Just Along For The Ride is a beautiful story of a mother and son's love for each other and the love of both for Christ. The sufficiency of God's grace in the most difficult time of life is an eternal truth experienced in a fresh and new way in the lives of these two beautiful people. You will be overwhelmingly blessed as you make the journey with them."

Dr. John Bisagno, Pastor Emeritus
Houston's First Baptist Church,
Speaker and Author

★   ★   ★

Anyone can benefit from reading about the all-too-brief life of Bill Roddy. It is at once inspiring, heartwarming, and humorous. Bill's story is a road map for anyone who desires to both give and receive the utmost from this life and, more importantly, throughout eternity. It would be a meaningful addition to any library.

Robert E. Driver, PhD
Professor of Finance and Ethics
LeTourneau University
April 21, 2011

★   ★   ★

NASCAR is a sport that rises and grows stronger in the face of adversity. This is the character of the sport and it is merely a reflection of the character of its fans . . . and Bill is a perfect example. Faced with adversity he chooses to move forward in life with faith, hope and love. His story as told by his mother will awaken within us all a desire to face challenges as Bill did . . . determined, focused and confident that God is in control. Those of us who are involved in NASCAR know the fans of this sport are what make it great . . . and Bill is one of the greatest!

Billy E. Mauldin, Jr., President and CEO
Motor Racing Outreach (MRO)

Just Along for the Ride

*The Amazing Journey of
William Baine Roddy*

MARTHA RODDY

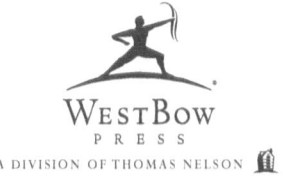

WESTBOW
PRESS
A DIVISION OF THOMAS NELSON

WestBow Press books may be ordered through booksellers or by contacting:

WestBow Press
A Division of Thomas Nelson
1663 Liberty Drive
Bloomington, IN 47403
www.westbowpress.com
1-(866) 928-1240

ISBN: 978-1-4497-3847-1 (hc)
ISBN: 978-1-4497-3848-8 (sc)
ISBN: 978-1-4497-3849-5 (e)
Library of Congress Control Number: 2012901467

Printed in the United States of America

WestBow Press rev. date: 03/09/2012

Contents

In memory of

my beloved husband,

Stephen Robert Roddy, MD, FACS;

our dearly loved son,

William Baine Roddy;

and our darling little angel,

Stephanie Renee Howard

Our loving

daughter-in-law and daughters,

Carrie,

Libby and Mary;

sons-in-law,

Jeff Rook and David Howard;

and our grandchildren,

Kyle, Josh, and Mason Rook,

Christopher and Amanda Roddy,

and Samantha and Andrea Howard,

and great-granddaughter,

Jayden Leslie Roddy

"Tell your children of it, and let your children tell their children, and their children another generation . . . Rejoice in the Lord their God" (Joel 1:3; 2:23).

"Before I formed thee in the belly, I knew thee; and before thou camest forth out of the womb I sanctified thee, and I ordained thee a prophet unto the nations" (Jeremiah 1:5).

Foreword

I became pastor of First Baptist Church, Port Charlotte, Florida, in 1965, and was impressed with the vitality and enthusiasm of a three-year-old church made up of mostly senior citizens. I was only thirty-one at the time, and those wonderful people took me, my wife, Gale, and our two small sons under their wings. Among the members, a young doctor and his wife made a huge impression on us. Dr. Stephen Roddy and his wife, Martha, were among those who welcomed us to Port Charlotte. They were very active in our church. Dr. Roddy became a deacon, and Martha served in numerous roles in the church.

It was amazing to watch the little Roddys, Libby, Bill, and Mary Seale, as they grew up.

Martha had them in church from the time they were born, and our nursery workers were happy to have them. Remember, we were living in a retirement community, so babies were a special blessing.

As the children grew, my middle son and Bill became close friends. Perhaps it was because they liked to have a good time and play tricks on others or just cause confusion for the pastor on occasions during the worship services. As they grew older, Bill and Steve would sit in the back row, and I wondered what they were getting out of the service. God works in mysterious ways, for Bill indicated early that he wanted to be a Christian. Much of his early learning about Jesus came from his home, which was as it should have been.

The Roddy family was a blessing to our church, and we experienced a profound loss when they chose to move to Texas. One would think that the distance between Florida and Texas would cause relationships to diminish to the point of forgetting, but not so with the Parkers and the Roddys, particularly, between Steve and Bill. Over the years, they remained best of friends and visited each other as often as possible. The bond of love between the two could only be broken by death. The reunion in heaven will be sweet for brothers and sisters in the Lord, and we all can look forward to seeing our Lord and Savior, Jesus, and our loved ones in God's beautiful heaven.

—Reverend John Parker, retired Director of Missions
Santa Fe River Baptist Association, Gainesville, Florida

Preface

On June 10, 2010, I began writing *Just Along for the Ride* for family and friends. In July, I presented the work-in-progress at a meeting of the Houston Inspirational Writers Alive! Several writer friends considered the spiritual message worthy of publication. Some suggested that in the wake of grief, the writing was therapeutic and healing for me. That may be true.

In my heart, I wrote to share Bill's faith and God's grace when cancer struck and to herald the vital need for early screening of cancer. My hypothesis is that the course of cancer parallels sin. Some sins are evident; other sins are unseen, silent predators that shatter human souls. Some cancers are visible; other cancers are hidden, mute pirates that wreck human bodies.

We all have the potential for sin. The good news is, know and apply God's Word to your life for He *restoreth* your soul. The same is true with colon cancer. We all have the potential for cancer. The good news, information, and technology are available to help prevent and cure some cancers, especially colon cancer. Early recognition of sin helps renew our spirit and hope; early detection of cancer helps to repair our bodies. God offers new hope each day for victims of sin; medical science tenders new hope each day for sufferers of cancer. Sin and cancer are universal. People face sin and disease each day. I do not believe that God causes sin or disease. I do believe that early detection of sin or cancer may prevent growth.

The courage to face cancer merits an award to every cancer patient. Most cancer victims are part of a medical team who contribute to medical science. Courageous cancer patients who endure pave the road for better health for all of us. Their bravery warrants gratitude and is an inspiration to fight for the prevention and cure of cancer.

Just Along for the Ride introduces my son Bill, who recognized that life holds multiple issues and he believed that cancer was only one of them. He knew he was in God's care and trusted God's will. He believed prevention, early screening, and a cure for cancer were within reach, but needed research money to achieve these goals.

Early detection serves both health and soul. Vigilance wins in life, whether it is a spiritual or physical battle. Bill met each day upbeat and aggressive, with a smile on his face, and a twinkle in his eye. My passion is to share Bill's happiness, hope, and faith. My prayer is to help you feel his Savior's gentle touch and to make it easier for you to smile and be filled with joy, whatever your circumstances.

I hope the chronicle of Bill's life sheds more light on the suffering and strength of people with colon cancer and *all* cancer—a disease that claims the lives of thousands of individuals every year.

If your life is free of disease or stress, may your soul prosper from learning about Bill Roddy's happy journey through life with God at his side.

Acknowledgments

My love is given to my daughters, Mary Howard and Libby Rook, for their help and consent to make this book happen. Mary's help with names and Libby's assistance scanning photographs and help with the cover were invaluable.

From the beginning, writer friends encouraged my efforts to publish *Just Along for the Ride*. My appreciation goes to Martha Rodgers, Wanda Shadle, Diana Battista, and others in Houston's Inspirational Writers Alive! (IWA!), as well as Melanie Stiles and those in DiAnn Mills' Wordsmith group in Houston, who critiqued and offered encouragement early in the writing. Mary Wade, friend and founder of Houston's Society of Children's Book Writers and Illustrators (SCBWI), freely gave of her expertise and skill for the manuscript-in-progress. I am grateful to Vicki Chapman, Beth Cross, Julie Herman, Linda Leschak, Heather Walters, Tina Wissner, Kathleen Endler, and members of the SCBWI critique group who met in my home and strengthened my efforts. Beth and Linda edited multiple pages of the manuscript on their own time.

Thanks to Roddy Noll and Harold Picton for their aeronautical expertise on landing gears of small planes and to Lori Robertson, who offered many a meal, while James

Robertson walked me through computer applications and scanned photographs. I appreciated Richard Talbot's interest in sharing the link to the *Houston Chronicle* article about the supercomputer IBM donated to Rice University for medical research.

Two wonderful friends, Betty Brandon from Punta Gorda, Florida, and Jean Ross, my college roommate from Pelahatchie, Mississippi, encouraged my efforts in writing this book. Delonda Delony, Michael Draper, and Bobby Plyler from San Marcos Baptist Academy Alumni, and Madeline De Long, director of SMA alumni office, and Amy Nighbert, SMA librarian, also helped tremendously in writing the book. I appreciate the interest of former SMA faculty members, Shella Baccus, teacher; Dr. Jimmy Cobb, chaplain; and Alan Hamlin, director of the SMA choir.

I am thankful for others who supported my efforts with the manuscript, including Brandon Burke, deacon, Houston's First Baptist Church; Reverend Larry Womack, pastor at Copperfield (Baptist) Church, Houston; Alana Smith, editor, *The Compass*, Copperfield Church senior newsletter; Paul Petropolis, sports writer and founder of Angels in Action, and Dr. Tommy Bambrick, Houston Baptist University, for his interest and help. Lori Roeckers, facilitator, WORDsearch Corporation, heartened my efforts to share my son's battle with cancer. I appreciated Edna Jane and Vernon Peeples, Punta Gorda, Florida, for their interest and Missy deSousa's, Public Affairs & Communication Project Manager, Motor Racing Outreach, for help with accuracy of information.

My gratitude goes to John Parker, Bill's lifelong pastor of Santa Fe River Baptist Association, Gainesville, Florida, who wrote the Foreword. I'll be forever refreshed in spirit remembering

Bill's pastors, Reverend Steve Washburn, Reverend John Woods, and Bill LaGrone, Adult Bible Fellowship teacher, First Baptist Church, Pflugerville, Texas, who supported Bill and his family and prayed with us throughout Bill's struggle with an unseen enemy. I will always remember Reverend Steve Washburn's words as he stood beside me before Bill's casket: "You know he is not there."

I am indebted and blessed with Nan Snipes, professional editor of *Just Along for the Ride*. My heartfelt thanks for the incredible editing of *Just Along for the Ride* goes to David Dunn, Diana K. Schramer, and other editors in the Westbow Press Editorial Department. Thank you to Jeremy Waddell, Sarah Goddard, Sam Fitzgerald, and WestBow Press; Graham van Dixhorn, author of *Write to Your Market*; Don Anders Photography; Rowe Ray, Managing Editor of *San Marcos Daily Record*; and others who graciously granted permission to use articles and photographs credited in the manuscript.

If I have omitted anyone's name, please forgive me. I am deeply moved by the encouragement, persuasion, and support of each individual who contributed their time and friendship.

Bill's Favorite Bible Verses

"And all things, whatsoever ye shall ask in prayer,
believing, ye shall receive them"
(Matthew 21:22).

"Now the God of hope fill you with all joy and peace
in believing, that ye may abound in hope,
through the power of the Holy Ghost"
(Romans 15:13).

"And the prayer of faith shall save the sick,
and the Lord shall raise him up;
and if he committed sins, they shall be forgiven him"
(James 5:15).

"And ye shall serve the Lord your God
and he shall bless thy bread, and thy water;
and I will take sickness away from the midst of thee"
(Exodus 23:25).

"Fear thou not; for I am with thee, be not dismayed; for I am
thy God: I will strengthen thee; yea, I will help thee; yea, I will
uphold thee with the right hand of my righteousness"
(Isaiah 41:10).

PRAYER

Stephen R. Roddy, MD

Lord, our Father, we thank Thee that in this day and time of the new theology, we have those who remain steadfast in the faith as revealed in Thy holy Word. We thank Thee for the assurance that there always will be those who will not be tossed about by the philosophies of man.

We thank Thee for revealing Thyself in the flesh that we might know Thee and for offering to us life in all fullness for which it was intended and for the honesty to reject or accept Thee.

For these things, we thank Thee in the abiding name of Christ.

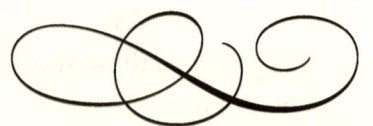

Chapter One
Never Felt Better

"I never felt better in my life, and now they are telling me I have colon cancer. I have to have surgery."

With a powerful note of certainty, my son's voice boomed over the telephone line, and his words pierced my heart with the force of a jagged thorn. I had expected the call from him about a colonoscopy scheduled that day, but the result of the procedure unnerved me and shattered the moment for me.

"A pathology report determines whether a mass is cancer or not, Bill," I offered in hope that the mass seen during the colonoscopy was benign.

"The gastroenterologist knew by looking at it, Mom. It's cancer," Bill countered.

Three months earlier, in April of 2009, Bill drove to a hospital in Austin, Texas, and staggered into the emergency room. Attendants threw him on a gurney and raced him into the operating room. In twenty-eight minutes, a surgeon had inserted two stents in his heart. Doctors determined that internal bleeding had contributed to a heart attack.

Several weeks before his heart attack, our family met for my birthday at Bill's house, and I was stunned to see him so devoid of color.

I spoke plainly, "You need to see a doctor, son. You look pale."

"I work inside and never see the sun, Mom. I'm okay."

After the birthday weekend, Bill's pale appearance remained a concern. When Carrie, Bill's wife, called saying Bill had a heart attack, it confirmed my fears. Jim Robertson, my neighbor, offered to drive, and we raced to Bill and Carrie's home in Pflugerville, Texas, close to St. David's North Austin Hospital.

When I saw Bill the next day, he looked much better than I'd seen him in March, and he felt good enough to hassle nurses and doctors about getting out of the hospital. Doctors knew the loss of blood helped trigger the heart attack. Scores of tests and several procedures ordered in the hospital failed to pinpoint the source of the internal bleeding, and doctors ruled out a colonoscopy following the emergency stent placement. Although Bill wanted to go home sooner, doctors ordered six blood transfusions before discharging him a week later.

Bill recovered quickly from the stent procedure and went back to his job. As soon as allowed by the doctor, he rode his bike every day after work. During the next few months, physicians continued to monitor him but found no evidence on laboratory reports of the source of his internal bleeding. Bill seemed assured that he was well and flew to Florida with his family for a planned July Fourth weekend.

The second week in August, evidence on laboratory tests substantiated bleeding from the colon. Disregarding the risk factor from the recent stent procedure, doctors ordered a colonoscopy.

After the initial shock of colon cancer found during Bill's colonoscopy procedure, my anxiety eased somewhat. I'd had several scares myself that involved tumors diagnosed as possible cancer. When I was twenty-eight, doctors found an obstructed colon, and I underwent a colectomy—the removal of a section of the colon. Much to my relief, the colon mass was benign.

In 2007, on routine examination, a physician discovered a mass in my abdomen, revealing the possibility of ovarian cancer. I sought a second opinion at M. D. Anderson. Helen E. Rhodes, M.D. at the MDA Gynecologic Oncology Center ordered blood work and a sonogram. The mass proved to be a cyst. Dr. Rhodes ordered follow-ups for the cyst and a colonoscopy—my first. My own assessment was that my health was great, and I didn't schedule the colonoscopy for months. I had the procedure shortly before my next appointment with Dr. Rhodes.

The delayed colonoscopy revealed a large polyp in the upper right colon that required surgery. For the second time in my life, I was scheduled for a colectomy for possible colon cancer. I debated if I even wanted to go through another colon resection and called Dr. Rhodes at MDA. An appointment for a second opinion at M. D. Anderson was set up with a surgeon, who ordered a repeat colonoscopy.

Bill and his daughter, Amanda, accompanied me to MDA for the colonoscopy. A skilled gastroenterologist, Patrick M. Lynch, M.D., successfully removed the large mass during the procedure. To my relief, the pathology report came back with the diagnosis of a precancerous polyp. I had avoided a second colon surgery, but I was guilty of assessing my own health and postponing a colonoscopy. I'd committed the unthinkable by delaying colon cancer screening.

When a polyp is removed before it has a chance to become malignant, the cure and survival rates are higher. I hoped the pathology report on the mass in Bill's colon would alleviate pressing fears less than a year after my own scare.

While discussing Bill's colonoscopy over the phone, he and I talked about my experiences. I had avoided surgery twice when I went to M. D. Anderson for a second opinion and treatment. I sensed that Bill had a positive attitude and pictured him squaring his broad shoulders in a military brace. His voice resounded with inner strength, as always. My son was a fighter. He tackled problems head-on. He never took a backseat when challenged, but I wasn't surprised at his closing remark, which was spoken in a less detached voice.

"It's in the Lord's hands, Mom. I'm just along for the ride."

From that moment on, Bill tackled his predicament with the zeal of a scientist. Almost dispassionately, he checked out statistics on colon cancer as well as the best hospitals and doctors in the United States for colon surgery.

Bill's pale face in March continued to nag at my mind. From my own experiences, I remained hopeful about his prognosis, and I prayed he would have a reprieve from cancer. His faith in God uplifted my spirits. I prayed for Bill's healing in God's grace and glory.

My son's large, bright blue eyes and smile were his trademark. Blond as a child, he was fair with a ruddy complexion. He had a muscular, athletic build. At six feet tall, his height came from a long, straight spine. He wore sport or dress coats well. No doubt I was prejudiced, but I thought he was handsome.

Bill rarely had a sick day at school or work. He would turn forty-six on August 22. He was such a happy soul. As I thought of my aggressive, robust son, another long-ago memory of a day in Gainesville, Florida, surfaced.

Chapter Two
Hello, World!

All babies are extraordinary. The first time I held my gangly infant in my arms, I kissed him. I felt my baby's warm body next to mine, and I knew I held the most extraordinary son ever in my arms.

When the time came to leave for home, I eased our newborn onto a padded table to change him into a take-home outfit bought in Fort Myers, Florida, especially for the occasion. At my touch, my amazing bundle of joy activated. Flinging and kicking, his gyrating limbs presented a challenge. My husband laughed at my ineptness and gently held down his son's appendages.

To meet her brother, I dressed our toddler in a pretty dress from the same Fort Myers baby boutique. Libby squeezed between Steve and me to help with her squirming sibling. Finally, dressed in a garment that was handmade in Switzerland and exquisitely embroidered with tiny elephants, giraffes, and tigers, our infant son was ready for his first ride home.

Steve settled our baby and me in the backseat of our Thunderbird® and put Libby in the front seat next to him.

Pleased to be promoted to the front seat, Libby readily accepted the baby in the carrier on the backseat.

That first night, I couldn't wait to lay our baby down to sleep in another handmade garment from Switzerland. He dozed off in a wisp of cotton—a miniature man's white nightshirt with edges trimmed in baby blue. Matching frogs, complicated braided cord fasteners, adorned the front of his nightdress. I stared in wonder at his little crimson feet and pulled booties over his tiny toes. I wrapped him in a soft blanket and placed our precious son in his crib. In minutes, I heard a loud cry. Kicking and screaming and out of the swaddling blanket, Bill had half-ripped the intricate frogs off the adorable infant nightshirt. That was the beginning of the end of his handmade baby clothes from Switzerland.

Our newborn was born active and strong. Within days, when I held him close to me, I felt his little arms tighten around my neck. One day I found him, fiery red, shaking in his crib. Thinking he was having a seizure, I yelled for the doctor, his father.

"Something is the matter with the baby!"

His dad ran to the crib and bent over at mattress level to check out his long, shaking-all-over son.

"Pick him up. Do something!"

My husband straightened up slowly, scratched his head, and said, "He's trying to push up."

"He's too young," I argued.

"Well, he's doing push-ups. There is nothing the matter with him."

Steve was right. Our happy, blond, blue-eyed baby was vigorous, tenacious—and determined. So began days filled with the unexpected, coupled with exuberant love, laughter, and blessings.

My husband took pride in naming each of the children. I named our first daughter Elizabeth Ann, Ann for my sister. Steve shortened her name to Libby. She called herself Libby Ann Dr. Roddy to her father's delight.

I wanted to name our son after his father, Stephen Robert Roddy III, but my husband had other ideas and chose William, his brother's name. Of old German origin, William delineated one a protector, supervisor, or overseer. William proved to be the perfect name for him. Steve added Baine of Scottish Gaelic origin and my maiden name, which means fair-haired and tall with strong bones. Not into the origin of names, we were unaware that our family names with Roddy, a good Irish surname, matched traits associated with German, Scottish, and Welsh heritage.

In French, the meaning of *bain* is bath. Baine was a harbinger for long soaks in the tub that later became a daily routine for our son. William Baine soon became Bill. Libby labeled her sibling Baby Bill until he threw the first punch at the belittling tag.

Fifteen months after Bill's arrival, our tiniest baby was born. Steve chose Martha Seale, my given name and my mother's maiden name, for our youngest daughter. I scotched that. I knew I would become Big Martha. Steve settled on Mary Seale, and I found the combination of the two names very pretty. In time, Mary Seale shortened her own name to Mary.

Libby and Bill greeted their new sister with excited pulls and tugs. Mary Seale's bottle became a snack for Libby and an object to throw for Bill. Our new baby screamed with terror at the sight of her siblings. Steve put a lock high on our bedroom door to protect our bald baby who had cotton-top sprigs of hair and twinkling eyes the color of a blue-green sea.

Chapter Three
Hanging Out Together

Our first wonderful experience with infants was with Libby. She gave up the two o'clock bottle ahead of schedule and her nights were predictable. Her cry was soft; her skin beautiful. She had no feeding problems. Content with a pacifier, she never put her thumb in her mouth. She laughed and cooed happily and won our hearts with sparkling eyes of denim-blue. She learned to talk early and enunciated clearly. She was good when I slipped little dresses over her blond curls. We prided ourselves on our parenting, not realizing that Libby's progress was innate and had nothing to do with our skills. We hovered over our daughter. One day, Steve decided we were spoiling our little princess. She needed a sibling.

The nursery scene changed upon the arrival of William Baine Roddy. He slept little, spit out pacifiers, pulled nipples off baby bottles, and hurled bottles across a room. His skin was sensitive to soap and fabrics. He blistered easily. Feeding him baby food proved a disaster. If he didn't like a jar of baby food—watch out! He spewed spinach all over the kitchen wall. He climbed out of his baby crib and landed on his bottom. He walked before I was ready.

Until Bill could put on his own clothes, he wrestled with anyone trying to dress him. During one of my daily struggles, Steve walked into the nursery, ushered me out, and closed the door. I heard all kinds of bumps and knocks coming from the room. Steve re-appeared with Bill in his arms. They had had a good workout. Father and son were red in the face and their clothes wet with perspiration.

A good-natured baby, Bill was quick as lightning. He chuckled and made all kinds of funny noises. I never anticipated his next move, and I was surprised and unnerved, on occasion, with his progress from one milestone to another.

He wouldn't take a pacifier but wanted his thumb. Determined, I'd pull his thumb out of his mouth, and just as determined, he'd pop his thumb right back in his little chops. Libby taught him with three quick smacks to his face not to put his thumb in his mouth. He yelled and yelled at Libby, but the thumb never touched his mouth again. With a little discipline, Bill was an apt learner.

These were the days before disposable diapers. Bill kicked and rolled over every time we changed him. Fortunately, I stuck myself with safety pins more than I did him. I became more frenzied each day trying to diaper Bill, and to solve my problem, my mother suggested putting him in training pants. He graduated far too early for training pants, but he liked pulling on his own "big boy" pants.

Shortly after Bill's advance to training pants, we were out and about on a Saturday afternoon in Fort Myers, Florida. I was always eager to go in Maas Brothers department store, and this was our first stop. In a concession to my husband, we strolled through the men's section. In seconds, Bill's actions caught our attention. We saw him vigorously scrubbing the floor. Our toddler had tinkled on the floor, and then grabbed a hat off a display to wipe up the puddle. Red-faced, Steve bought the hat, and we left Maas in a hurry for home. Maybe that was the beginning of Bill's obsession with clean floors.

Bill began to talk, and no one understood him but me. I hauled him off to a speech therapist. The speech therapist engaged me in conversation and quickly diagnosed the cause of Bill's unintelligible speech—his mother.

"He is mimicking you. You speak rapidly and swallow beginning and ending sounds. Speak slowly and clearly for a week. That will clear up your son's speech."

In a week, Bill's jumbled words disappeared. His deep and expressive voice as a toddler developed into a mature voice, full of meaning and an unforgettable resonance. As an adult, he was as articulate as the best of speakers.

Our children matured faster than we could keep up. We were never ready for their increasing mobility and actions.

Before the children were born, we bought a house on a canal that widened into a lagoon in back of the property. The great location on the water presented hazards for young children. We wanted to stay on the water and decided to enclose a safe play area off the patio for them. After much discussion, we signed a contract with a contractor who designed a costly structure to withstand hurricane-force winds, a fence to prevent the children from climbing.

Libby and Bill loved the added freedom of walking out the patio door onto the grass to play. The safe play lasted less than a week. I couldn't turn my back on the two of them to take care of the baby. Bill climbed the fence, and they dug a large hole at the edge of the patio.

"Martha, put this house on the market," Steve said. "We've got to get out of here. The ink wasn't dry on the contractor's check before Bill climbed that fence. Now, look at them. They're digging a swimming pool out there."

Obviously, they were capable of digging under the fence. We moved to the country to give the children a safe place to play. One day in a Florida setting sun, I noticed the light seemed to shine through Bill's fair skin. He appeared translucent, an angelic moment I never forgot.

As the years passed, we enjoyed the children's different personalities and watched them relate to each other. Bill developed significant relationships with his sisters. He kept an eye on Libby. Libby learned to write her name early and penned her name on pages of the family Bible. Bill wanted to write his name too. We found a "B" and three sticks written on numerous pages of the Bible. Scribbling in books was forbidden, but I treasured their signatures in our family Bible. I never dreamed I'd see a "B" and three sticks incised on an open Holy Bible on a granite marker.

There were few confrontations between the girls and Bill. They were no match for his strength. Even though they became angry with him at times, his sisters adored their energetic and fun brother.

Libby and Bill played well together, and he lived up to the name William. In Chattanooga at Evelyn's, Steve's sister, we witnessed Bill in a hilarious scene. After a boy teased Libby, her brother went into action. With a stick resembling a harpoon, Bill raced after the older lad, who ran up and down and over a hill to avoid a walloping strike from our son.

Equally protective of Mary, Bill's relationship with his younger sister was different. He not only protected, he supervised her. A little imp, Mary was a care for her brother. He ran or climbed after his little sister to keep her out of harm's way.

One day, I overheard Bill's stern voice. "You listen to me. You do what I say. When Daddy's gone, I'm the daddy."

Mary never forgot his line. In college, whenever she ran out of money, she ran to her brother.

★   ★   ★

Life for our small children advanced from home to community. They were all set to go out into the world, but I'm not sure we were.

In the sixties, no seat belts existed in cars, and I drove alone with three young children, sitting in the backseat, untethered. On trips to town, we had to cross railroad tracks. Once, I stopped the car at a railroad crossing, and an impatient driver in the car behind our Oldsmobile® honked so I would hurry across. In the rearview mirror, I caught a glimpse of Bill shaking a fist at the man.

I scolded him, "Wait until your father hears that you shook your fist at that man."

After my account of his son's actions, I expected Steve at least to reinforce with a father-son talk. It didn't happen. Instead, Steve grinned. An obvious father-son bond existed.

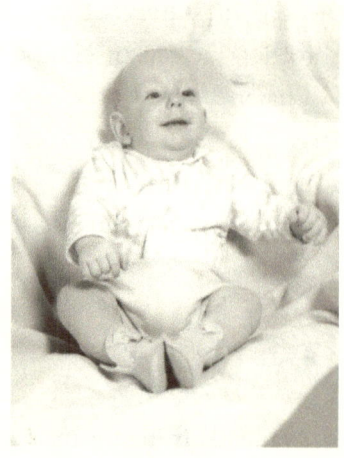

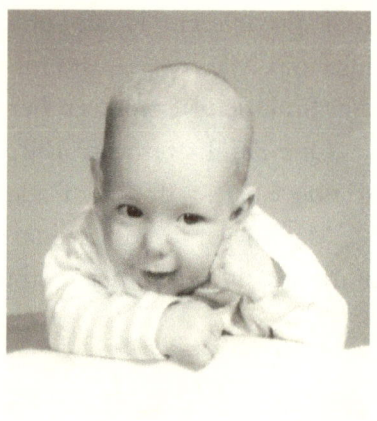

A happy baby   I'm thinking tricks

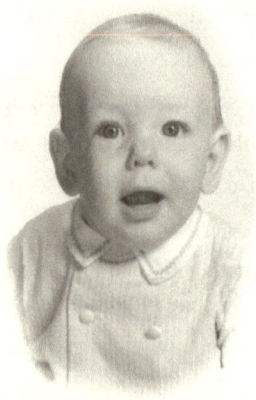

I'm ready to go!
William Baine Roddy

Toddlers Two

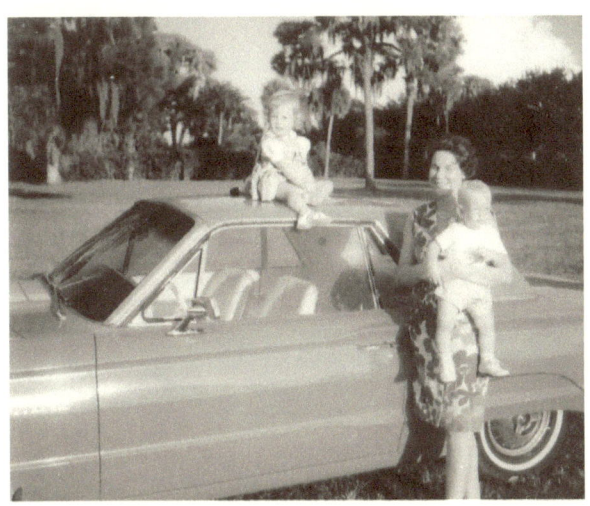

This is a bummer

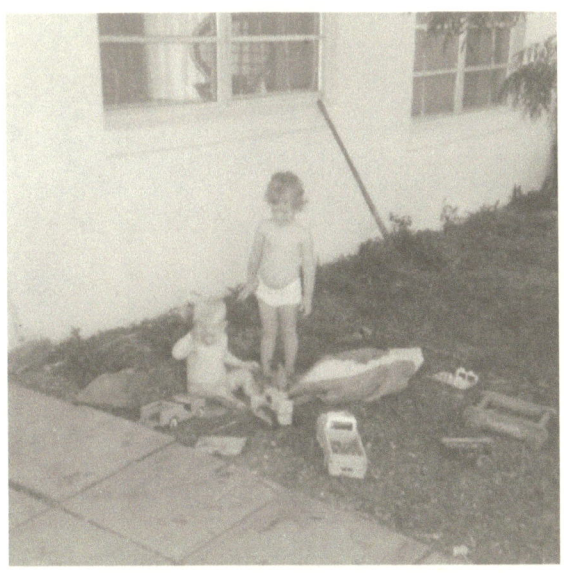

Digging a swimming pool for two

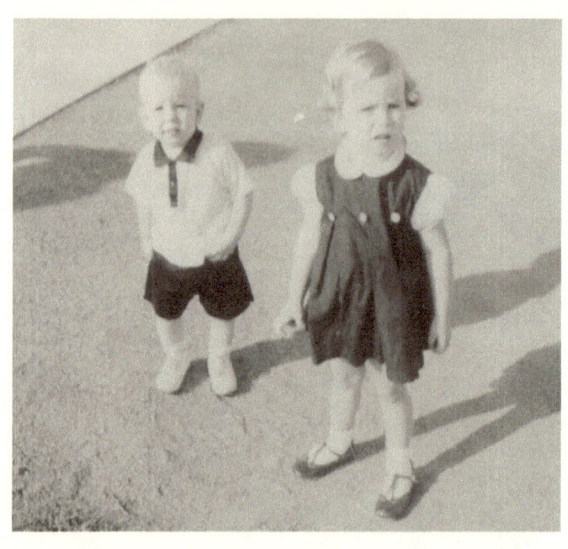

Serious trouble—caught in the street
Bill and Libby

Now We are Three

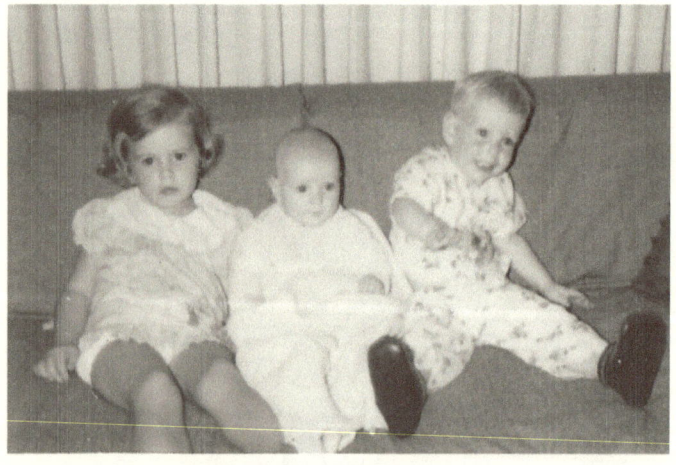

Cameras are for girls, not me!
Libby, Mary, and Bill

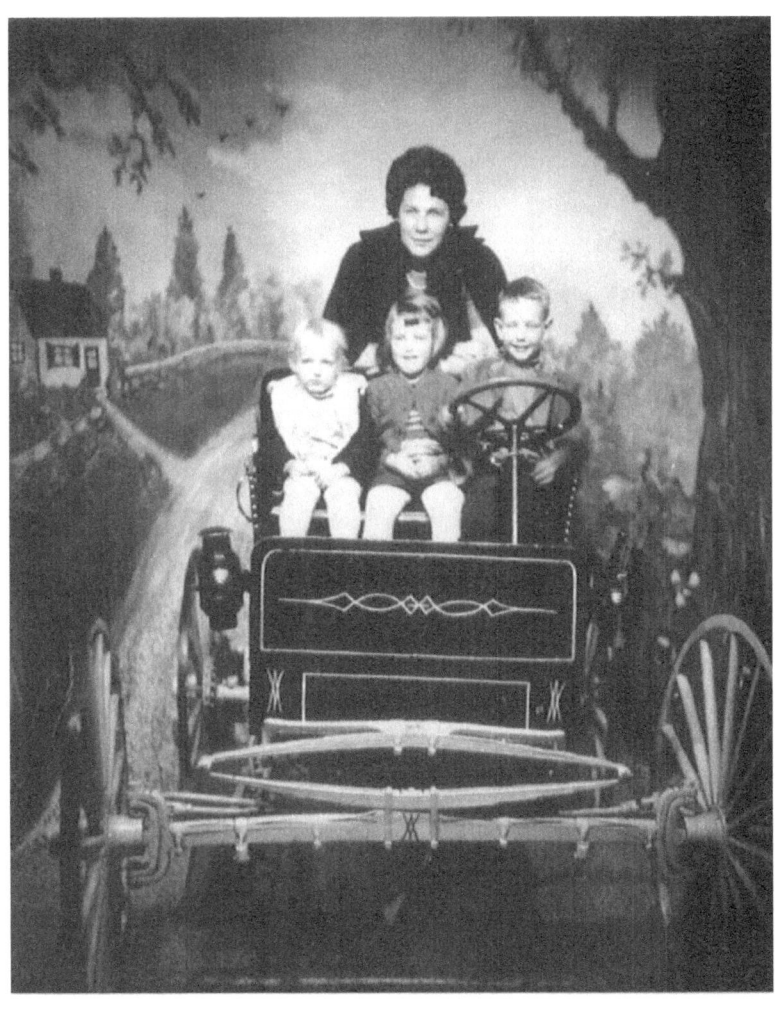

Mary, Libby, Bill, and Martha
Chicago Museum of Science and Industry 1968
CMSI Yesteryear Photo

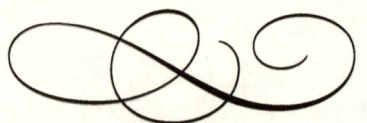

Chapter Four
Profession of Faith

Bill's ability to read people proved advanced for his age. On a trip to the mall, Santa asked Bill what he wanted for Christmas. Bill pressed his lips together and refused to talk.

Later, I asked him, "Why didn't you tell Santa what you wanted for Christmas?"

"He's nothin' but a clown."

Although his comment seemed an uncanny reply for someone only three years old, Bill's take on Santa was a forerunner of his insight. Man created the man in red, a brilliant idea, but Bill didn't buy it. He had a natural ability to see clearly and intuitively into the complexity of a person, situation, or subject. That December day, I failed to see what that meant in God's plan for his life.

In our church, four was the customary age for a child to be in worship services. "Bill is four now," I reminded Reverend Parker, "and it's time for him to attend "big church" services."

"You don't need to rush it, Martha," he said.

Reverend Parker knew the score with four-year-old boys in the sanctuary—he had three young sons, Timothy, Stephen, and

Jonathan. Against John's pastoral advice, I chose to take Bill into the most sacred service in our church.

At the close of the worship services in southern Baptist churches, the minister invites those in the congregation to come forward. Requests vary for those who walk to the front of a Baptist church. Some church members want to move membership from another Baptist church. For others, the invitation offers a refuge to request prayer. Most important, the invitation gives the unsaved participant the opportunity to declare his or her love and belief in Jesus Christ and ask for forgiveness of sins. A profession of faith, the commitment to Jesus for salvation and everlasting life, is followed by baptism and church membership.

Bill was all eyes and ears during the first few Sundays in the sanctuary. He enjoyed pulling the hymn book out of the rack and turning the pages. Musical by nature, he loved to sing. He'd glance at the hymnal in my hands, and then examine the hymnal in his hands. He recognized the dissimilarity of the pages in his hymnal and mine and wanted his book to match mine. With a teaching background, I beamed that he'd grasped the difference in the hymn books. He could read. I came to realize later it was more than reading; it was a yearning to do things right. If he set his mind on something, he wanted to be on the right page.

Several Sundays into Bill's initiation to the worship service, following the closing prayer and invitation, I opened my eyes to find Bill gone. He'd disappeared from my side. I couldn't see over the heads of the standing congregation. Perplexed, I looked under the pew.

Then I heard our pastor. "Bill Roddy, we know you love Jesus. Now, go back up the aisle to your mother."

Thus began a struggle at the close of services on Sunday morning. I'd hold onto Bill during the invitation. At times during his first year in the sanctuary, he'd break away and run to the front of the church to the pastor.

One day, John called, "The next time Bill comes to the front to make his commitment, I plan to recommend him for baptism and church membership. I've questioned him. I've talked with him. I've prayed with him. He has reached the age of accountability. He understands what he is doing. He believes in John 3:16, in Jesus, and his own salvation and everlasting life. I don't want to keep turning him away."

Bill made a profession of faith, was baptized, and joined First Baptist Church in Port Charlotte, Florida, at the age of five. He wanted to be on the right page with Jesus.

Bill didn't believe in Santa Claus. He knew Jesus was for real.

Chapter Five
School Bells

Libby began a pre-kindergarten program in the Parish Day School sponsored by the Church of the Good Shepherd in Punta Gorda, and we had another struggle with Bill. When we arrived at the school, he wanted to go with Libby.

"You cannot go to kindergarten until you are older," I said. "We'll go to the park and play."

"No. Don't want to go to the park. I wanna go to school."

It was a daily battle. We enrolled our strong-minded son in the Episcopal pre-kindergarten program as soon as they'd accept him.

Bill loved the outdoors, but his fair skin burned in the sun. We kept him inside until late each day, and he had free reign to play in the house. Our son had not anticipated the staying inside and sitting in a chair regimen at school. He bucked the teachers. After one of his non-cooperative episodes, I called Steve at work about Bill's behavior. We had debated sending Bill off to school at four. He was getting off on the wrong foot at Good Shepherd. After my call, Steve arrived at the house, unannounced, to discipline Bill.

The next day in the grocery, a patient of Steve's walked up to me.

"I was in your husband's office yesterday. The nurse announced in the waiting room the doctor had an emergency and told us not to leave; he'd be back shortly. He sure left there in a hurry. Do you know what happened?"

I blinked at the question. I never knew the comings and goings of my husband with his patients and the hospital. I didn't want to know, so I could honestly say I wasn't aware of privileged information between the doctor and a patient.

"Well, must have been something terrible for him to hurry out of there like that," she said. "I thought you might know, Martha."

"Really?"

I did not answer her question. Family relationships are privileged information too. Dad's showing up unexpectedly to discipline Bill was the beginning of his settling down in pre-K and learning to conform under the regimentation of his teachers. Mrs. Goddard taught kindergarten in England prior to her position in the Church of the Good Shepherd, and Miss Hartnagle was an equally fine teacher. Both helped mold our growing son.

Steve scheduled a month off from his practice during Bill's kindergarten year and Libby's first year in school to take the second half of the American Board of Surgery exam for certification. The examination was to be held at the Medical College of Georgia/ University of Georgia in Augusta. Steve rented an apartment and insisted I pack up to go with him for the month of October. Bill and Libby had been in school for only a month, and I had reservations about pulling them out of school. We prayed that Libby and Bill would benefit from the challenge.

First Baptist Church in Augusta sponsored a school that answered our need. The first Monday we were in Augusta, we enrolled Libby and Bill in school at First Baptist. We settled into a nice three-bedroom apartment. Steve set up a study in one bedroom and closed the door to prepare for his board certification.

The first full day of school proved to be eventful. We left Libby and Bill at the school, and after returning to the apartment, I found Mary playing with a bottle of prescription pills.

I interrupted Steve to show him the bottle.

"Where did she get this?" he asked, reaching for Mary.

"I don't know," I said.

Steve grabbed Mary's pulse. "Have you taken any of these pills?"

She shook her head at the question, and then said, "Libby did."

"Mary's pulse is okay. I don't believe she's taken any of these pills. How long was she playing with the bottle, Martha?"

Steve continued taking Mary's pulse, without missing a beat, and alternated between that and checking her out.

"I don't know. When we took Libby and Bill to school, I didn't see Mary with the pills in the car. I'd only been in the kitchen a few minutes when I saw her with the bottle. Before we left the house this morning, Libby complained her head was hurting. I thought her headache was all about the new school."

"I can't believe Libby took the pills," he said. "She'd ask me first. If she did take them, they would kill her. I can't chance it."

Steve called the school, and we raced to our daughter while he continued checking Mary's pulse and questioning her.

"Where did you find this bottle, Mary?" he asked again.

"Baffroom," our three-year-old said softly.

"Where did you find them in the bathroom? The medicine cabinet?"

Mary nodded. "Libby did it."

At the school, we found Libby, bewildered and frightened, beside an ambulance, and surrounded by police. She burst into tears when she saw us. Steve grabbed her wrist to check her pulse while paramedics rattled off Libby's stats.

"Pulse normal," an ashen Steve said to me, wrapping his arms around our weeping Libby, as he continued to check both of the girls.

We tried to comfort Libby, but the crying continued. She couldn't understand why she was singled out by paramedics and police. Steve tried to explain, but she couldn't comprehend why he did such a thing.

"You did it, Daddy? You called them?"

Nothing we said helped Libby understand. In her mind, her parents instigated the whole scenario. We stayed at the school awhile to soothe our distraught daughter.

The day we moved into the apartment, I checked the medicine cabinets and Steve double-checked them. We later learned that the previous apartment renter searched without success for his missing bottle of heart medicine. He thought he'd accidentally knocked the bottle into the wastebasket and tossed it in the trash can. Mary saw us searching the medicine cabinets. A born climber, she went on her own little treasure hunt. Only her tiny fingers could have discovered the bottle nestled in a metal support adjacent to the medicine cabinet door. While getting the two older children off to school, I'd failed to keep a close eye on Mary. I trembled thinking how quickly a day can turn into a disaster with young children.

Thankfully, she didn't take any of the pills and neither, of course, did Libby.

That night at bath time, I was shocked to see red welts across Bill's back. He'd been in his first fight during recess, and his teacher was unaware of what had happened. We never knew what took place on the playground that day, but Bill wasn't afraid to go back to school.

The Roddys had arrived in Augusta, and, just as I feared, things weren't going well. My eyes filled with tears thinking about our sweet, frightened three-year-old and our innocent, terrorized Libby snatched by the police. Bill's fight at school concerned me. He was large for his age, and he did not balk about going back to the school. I assumed he won the fight. There could be more fights, and I didn't want to see any more welts on my young son.

Emotionally, after the day's experiences, the children were more stalwart than their mother. I was grateful that the Lord watched over them, but I was ready to leave Augusta. It would be easier for me to watch them at home.

"Nothing is as important as our children. I can't stay here with three children, Steve," I said. "We're going home."

Steve didn't give in easily. He promised to take a break in the afternoons to be with the children, an unheard of opportunity with his busy schedule at home.

The children and I stayed in Augusta, but my apprehension continued. I checked the children daily for signs of stress. Late one day, I looked out the apartment window to check on Bill.

I called out to Steve, "I'm going downstairs to get Bill. He's playing with boys who are much older than he is. I don't want him to get hurt."

Steve walked over to the window and watched Bill run with the football.

"They don't want him out there any more than you do. They throw the ball, and he runs out in front to catch it. He's in their way. Look at him! He's all over the place out there."

After our month in Augusta, Libby returned to East Elementary in Punta Gorda, and her teacher found her ahead in reading and math. Bill went back to Parish Day School kindergarten with no ill effects. We were grateful our children easily and quickly adapted to the change, and Steve successfully completed his boards. Overall, Augusta proved a positive experience for our family.

Bill's late-August birthday created concern about his entering first grade. I thought Bill, large for his age at six years and a few days, was too young and too active for first grade. I consulted with Mrs. Goddard. He passed the pre-first-grade tests with flying colors, and Mrs. Goddard found him one of the most self-sufficient children she'd ever taught. He was ready for first grade. Now I understood that when he'd ripped out of his infant nightshirt, pushed up in his crib, fought anyone who tried to dress him, and walked and talked early, he was expressing his self-sufficiency. The qualities of determination and confidence were evident from the beginning of his life.

Damaged by Hurricane Charlie, a larger, very different school now stands on the site where our children attended elementary school. The architectural design of the East Elementary we knew resembled a flower with wide-opened petals, a plan that won recognition and accolades in school architecture. Bill had waited impatiently for a year, watching Libby get out of the car and walk into the unique school. The day he entered first grade, there were no tears. He bubbled with enthusiasm as I walked with him along open-to-the-sky corridors to his class. The brightly decorated room, the teacher, and his classmates met his needs. He never glanced back at me.

The class voted Bill to be president of the first grade. In that role, he banged the gavel and called for order. As far as I know, this was the only political office he ever held. He was a people person, and my spirited, active son was on his way. I could never hold him back.

An early riser, Bill began his day in the middle of the night. Steve would come in from surgery in the wee hours of the morning and find Bill in the bathtub with water up to his ears. He feared Bill would fall asleep and drown.

"Martha, you have to watch him. Keep him out of that tub in the middle of the night."

"In the middle of the night?"

"In the middle of the night, Martha."

I wondered how I could keep an eye on Bill when I was sound asleep. Sometimes, Bill tried to get me up.

"It's not time to get up," I grumbled. "Go back to bed."

"No, I wanna see the sun come up."

One elementary school project—burying seeds in soil in a paper cup—motivated Bill to plant a garden. He worked and worked in chunky dirt to form straight and even rows. Our little farmer didn't like vegetables, but was thrilled at the sight of green sprouts that popped up in the garden.

Once, in the middle of the night, I heard, "Mama, get up."

Without opening my eyes, I urged with the usual, "Go back to bed, Bill. It's not time to get up. Go back to bed."

"You gotta get up. There's a skunk in my garden, and you have to help get him out." Apparently, his self-sufficiency didn't include skunks.

Edging out from under our wings at church, Bill tried sitting with Stephen Parker, the pastor's son, in a pew of their own choosing—at the back of the church.

One Sunday, we heard John Parker in a matter-of-fact tone of voice say from the pulpit, "Bill Roddy and Stephen Parker, come down here and sit in the front row." They learned that misbehavior in Sunday school and church wasn't without discipline by their wise pastor.

Sometimes, I received a call from Pastor Parker. "Have Bill at the church at eight o'clock on Saturday morning. I want Bill and Stephen to clean up the church yard."

Bill had fun at home, school, and church. His faith was real, and the inclination to write notes and his zeal for God carried over into his school assignments.

Put It in Writing

Written Messages Save Time and Eliminate Errors

Date 12-13 73

To Class Book

Subject Christmas

The star that led the Wise Men
to Christ's birthplace has fascin-
ated men throughout the ages.
In this handsome book, Franklyn
Branley tells the story of the
Wise Men's journey and
discusses the theory that our
astronomers have advanced
about this guide.

STANDARD FORM 113

Signed Bri Bill Robi.

Bill brought God to school.

The stellar study of the Star of Bethlehem in the 1966 edition of *The Christmas Sky* by Franklyn Mansfield Branley and the woodcut illustrations in subdued colors by Blain Lent captivated Bill's interest. In 1990, the publisher, Thomas Y. Crowell, New York, published a second edition of *The Christmas Sky* with beautifully colored illustrations by Stephen Fieser.

Bill's days of mischief coupled with imagination and ingenuity centered on wide-open spaces and the sky. After a trip to town, I entered our drive and caught sight of boards nailed on the towering Australian pine in the side yard. I knew who built the stairway to the stars, but I could not imagine where he acquired the lumber. I later found out. Bill's bed was in good condition when I left the house, but while I was gone, he had pulled the slats from under the springs and repositioned the springs and mattress on the floor within the bed frame. The sitter didn't realize the busy project at the tree involved bed slats from his bed. Bill's goal was to build a tree house. We settled the high-rise project with a stern warning—no more lumber from the house!

Pine needles and hard nut-like fruit covered the ground under the fast-growing Australian pine with a shallow root system. It was a nuisance to keep the new growth of little trees cleared out from under the tree. In truth, the tree, not a member of the pine family, wasn't safe for a playhouse and was much too tall for a castle in the sky.

The tree meant more to Bill than I ever realized. I found a poem, "My Favorite Tree," by Bill Roddy, unedited, left years ago in a chest in my house.

My Favorite Tree
by Bill Roddy

My favorite tree
is the Australian pine
growing on our property line.

This great tree
is very, very tall
and wide, wide, wide,
Because little trees
come up on every side.

The wind whistles through
its needles at night;
The tree stands great
with a lot of force and might.

I'd like to be like this tree
growing tall in the sky
And learn to withstand life's blows
with all.

I'd like to do something
to help others grow
And learn to help meet
the world's foe.

Long before his birthday, Bill would make a list of party
"to-dos" for me. This list included names of friends to invite,
Pin the Tail on the Donkey for fun, and ice cream and cake

with candles. Steve was appalled that I'd let our birthday boy and girls blow out candles on a cake, and then serve their guests a slice of germs.

Germs on birthday cakes were the least of my worries. I was more concerned with the children's table manners. Steve worked long hours and seldom made it home in time for dinner with the children. We scheduled family dinner at home after church on Sunday. Steve kept the children at the table while he read the Bible and taught tenants of the Old and New Testaments.

Hospital or patient calls delayed many a Sunday meal. I insisted the children wait at the table to eat until their father sat down and said the blessing. Waiting to eat gave time for instruction in table manners. One Sunday dinner is memorable.

"Don't touch the food on your plate until Daddy sits down. Practice chewing with your mouth closed. Don't put your elbows on the table, don't lick your fingers—use your napkin and keep one hand in your lap."

With one hand hidden under the table, Bill moved to grab a morsel off Mary's plate.

Mary reacted swiftly by stabbing Bill's wandering hand with her fork.

"Well, you said not to eat anything off *your* plate. Bill's eating off *my* plate, Mama."

Steve walked into the dining room to find his son's hand bleeding and hustled Bill off for peroxide, triple antibiotics, a bandage, and an added delay for Sunday dinner.

It was tough to wait until their dad sat down to eat, but our children learned at the dinner table that lessons and work come before pleasure. If you have a job, do your best and don't quit until the work is done. Steve's Bible lessons and work ethic were imprinted on their young minds. In their adult lives, they have worked hard and honored God's holy Word.

A few wrinkles were added to our brows on school days.

One morning, someone from school called and said, "Bill arrived at school in clothes that are in shreds. No other child in school looks as bad as he does."

It took awhile to figure out what happened. Temporary and impoverished agricultural workers' children rode our school bus. Some of the children wore tattered and torn clothing. In compassion, Bill had cut up good school clothes to look ragged so that he matched the attire of his friends on the bus. He stashed his cut-up outfit in a hole that he dug at the bus stop. Almost always first at the bus stop, he changed into clothes of his own design to wear to school. Bill's originals were overkill, and the school wanted him out of them.

I don't know if Bill attempted to make his needy friends feel better or if he liked the look of their clothes. Knowing Bill, both empathy and design played into his motives. Now, I see Bill originals (jeans full of holes) for sale everywhere in clothing stores.

Bill felt sympathy for needy animals as well as disadvantaged children. He fed steak planned for dinner once to a flea-infested, mangy, stray hound dog.

"You're not keeping that dog," I told him.

Bill was heartbroken when I called the dogcatcher, but I ignored his pleas. Evidently, Bill established a bond with the man who took the dog away because, five days later, the phone rang.

"Mrs. Roddy, the dog I picked up at your house is a nice, gentle dog, and it would be great for your children. I hate to put her to sleep."

I'd never been a supporter of euthanasia, so I agreed to take the dog. The moment the dog saw Bill, she jumped out of the truck, into his arms, and licked him for all she was worth. Coffee became a part of our family.

The next episode with Bill and animals involved a very pregnant stray cat.

"You cannot keep that cat, son."

"I'm keeping this cat; she is going to have kittens."

Surprised that he figured that out at his age, I gave in to Bill. We kept the cat.

Fortunately, her birthing time occurred during one of my Saturday afternoon trips to the grocery. Steve was at home, and I'm sure only one in a million cats delivers eight kittens with a board-certified surgeon in attendance. Steve remarked that he was first assistant to Bill, who was already on the case, excitedly supervising each of the eight deliveries. To him, each kitten was a miracle. Bill learned the facts of life from his dad that day. As long as we lived in the country, we had a yard full of cats originating from that first litter.

Busy with his practice until late evening and often working at night, Steve wanted and counted on Bill and the girls to help me at home. During WWII, he served in the US Army Air Force and had initiated a work program at home that reflected his military background. The girls resented the "orders" that Steve placed on the refrigerator for them, but Bill took the male responsibility seriously.

About the time Steve's work schedule appeared on the fridge, Bill's teacher gave an assignment for students to analyze the division of work and breakdown of family chores in the home. Bill was prepared. His chart was hilarious, and the totals brought laughs at school and home:

Father	Mother	Bill	Libby	Mary
0	2	20	1	0

Chapter Six
The Making of a Man

It is not my intent to paint a perfect family or a perfect son. We were average parents, at best. In our hearts, our children were the greatest in the world. Just as in your family, each child was different, an individual with a uniqueness of his or her own. Bill's traits often surprised us. He wasn't fearful, but he was cautious. He looked before he rounded a corner.

Once, while Bill was in middle school, his principal asked us to report to the school. Steve was furious that Bill had gotten into something at school that necessitated his absence from work. When we walked into his office, the principal handed us a letter detailing the authority to expel Bill for a fight at school. The principal said that Bill and his friends announced and advertised the upcoming fight all day in school, and a large crowd of students gathered after school to witness the event. We experienced the disappointing moment as graciously as possible and resolved to accept the decision and the punishment for his fighting at school.

Bill had no intention of accepting the decision to leave his world—school. "Sir, the fight wasn't at the school."

"What do you mean the fight wasn't at school?" the principal demanded.

"It wasn't on the school grounds. We made sure of that. We told everyone it would be after school in the street that runs between the middle school and the high school."

"What you don't know, Bill, is the school owns the street between the two campuses. The street is school property."

"I didn't know that, sir. We told everyone the fight would be after school, in the street, not on the school grounds."

The principal frowned and paused to give Bill's statement some thought. Bill's attitude and rationalization to fight in the street put a wrinkle in expulsion for a fight on campus. Obviously, Bill's intent to exchange physical blows centered on an off-campus fight. The principal gave the fighters the benefit of the doubt. To our relief, the two boys were not expelled. It was a close call. Bill had a way of landing on his feet.

Our son wasn't contentious. He didn't pick fights, and he didn't rush into them. He'd settle a discord. He never backed down. He'd look after someone who couldn't defend himself. Back at home, Bill's explanation for the fight was that his opponent threw his weight around at school. We were quick to tell him it wasn't his responsibility to settle issues at school by fighting.

In the aftermath of the fight at school, Bill came home pleased to tell us he was working for the principal. We assumed the job was subtle punishment for the fight and so the principal could keep an eye on our son. Bill showed the principal he liked to work, his aptitude and ability to do well. The principal, who became Bill's advocate, let us know Bill did an excellent job working for him in the front office.

Order seemed to come naturally to Bill. I don't remember getting after him to clean up his room. He had a built-in time clock. We never had to drag him out of bed for school or church. He dressed and impatiently waited on the rest of us. When he was older, if a night out came up, we'd agree on the time to come home. Bill never came home late. Time was synonymous to order with him.

Participation in an Amateur Athletic Union (AAU) swim program was the only sports activity the children shared. Our family enjoyed AAU swim meets in Gainesville, Orlando, and Fort Myers, but the children's other interests were different.

Bill had a passion for sports. He excelled on a school golf team. Little League and Punt, Pass, and Kick (PPK) trophies testified to his energy and enthusiasm for baseball and football. We sat in the bleachers, clapping and yelling for our young athlete who delighted in knocking a baseball over the fence.

"Did you see that?" his father said proudly, but he worried Bill would ruin his pitching arm in Little League games.

As a team player with a zeal for the rough and tumble, punting, passing, and kicking, football was our son's favorite sport. With Bill's dedication to sports, his father wanted to see serious study and enrolled him for his freshman year at nearby Bishop Verot Catholic High School in Fort Myers, Florida. Bill played on the football team.

Another poem, unedited, from a *Journal of Poetry*, found in the chest at my house, speaks for itself about his love for football.

Bear Bryant
by
Bill Roddy

I have a hero whose
name is Bear.
He lives in Alabama,
but I've never been there.

I want to play football
for this famous man and
to reach this goal
I ran, ran, ran, but

I need a lot better grade in
English at Verot,
If I am ever to meet my hero.

The summer of 1979, we moved to Texas. For the next three years, Bill played football at San Marcos Baptist Academy (SMA). In the 1981 SMA yearbook, The Crest, Bill is listed on the varsity football team and was co-captain of the 1981 team. Jean Shand's book, *Echoes in Your Memories of San Marcos Baptist Academy*, 1990, lists Bill as an All-State player for 1980 and 1981, his senior year.

The San Marcos Academy football team went to the finals in 1980. Bill and Randy Brotherton were the only returning varsity football players in 1981, and they faced a dismal season with a team of younger players.

In the October 4, 1981, *San Marcos Daily Record* article, "Seniors Shoulder Academy Load," Sports Editor Russell Smith quoted Bill. "'I think what we're going through now just means that we've got to be leaders now; more even than we have in the past.'" According to Smith, Roddy and Brotherton couldn't have played any better in a recent game against Holy Cross. "Roddy, for example, turned in a sensational 18-tackle, six-sack performance . . . and Brotherton has been a mainstay on both offense and defense all season," he wrote.

In the same article, Smith referred to Bill as a 6-0, 200-pound nose guard, who expressed Frank Merriwellesque sentiments when he said, "'We consider it . . . as our duty, I guess.'" The sports editor said that as Bill spoke, "his friendly, open face showed no trace of bitterness about his team's fate, and there was no hint of irony in his voice."

When I re-read the yellowed newspaper article, I asked myself, "Why would a sports writer compare Bill Roddy to a Frank Merriwell?" I discovered that Frank Merriwell was a fictional hero created by Gilbert Patten under the pseudonym of Burt Standish. The Frank Merriwell series, published as early as 1904 in novels and short stories, later emerged in radio serials and comic books.

Frank Merriwell, a remarkable, make-believe athlete, with a merry disposition and a thriving vitality, deciphered mysteries and righted wrongs. He engaged in sports and received traumatic blows without injury. Loyal and brave, with a stoic mindset that served him well, Frank played in a world of sports filled with fun and thrills.

Russell Smith's comparison of Bill to Frank Merriwell was indeed an acute observation. Bill's sunny disposition warmed us day after day. His insight helped him decipher and solve problems and right wrongs. My husband mentioned Bill's threshold for pain from the time he was a baby. If he fell, he didn't cry; if knocked down, he jumped up. He kept going after hard blows, the kind that left Bill with a broken shoulder and injuries to both shoulders. Shoulder surgery in high school ended Bill's football career.

Twenty-nine years after Russell Smith's article, Bill Roddy faced a Frank Merriwell year with a demeanor almost fictional. Bill was not imaginary; he was real. In a seven-month battle with cancer, he approached life each day upbeat and ready to go for it.

San Marcos Baptist Academy groomed students for crises in life, Frank Merriwell-type predicaments. On a school trip, a potential disaster occurred in the presence of SMA students. Mary and Bill had traveled with the choir to Washington where the choir sang under the direction of Alan Hamlin at the Pentagon, National Cathedral, and Mount Vernon. For their return trip home, the SMA choir entered Dulles airport about the same time the US government deported Iranian diplomats and staff. When a crowd in the airport sneered and hurled insults at the deportees, the SMA choir spontaneously broke into Irving Berlin's "God Bless America." The media credited the choir with quelling a crisis at the airport. The incident spoke well for the school that helped mold teenagers into thoughtful, caring, patriotic young adults.

Our children were blessed with school and church activities that shaped character. On a high school mission trip, Bill went with a group to witness on a beach on Florida's east coast. Bill wasn't forward with people, but he wasn't shy either.

After the mission trip, I questioned Bill. "What did you say when you walked up to witness to a person on the beach?"

"Got a minute?" he asked.

I have a vivid memory of Bill at the front of the sanctuary, sharing the beach mission trip with those in church. At ease in front of the congregation, he spoke with an expressive tone of voice, which was truly a gift of God.

We counted our blessings. There was never a dull day with our children. The funny, the good, and the love mirror the happy days in my heart.

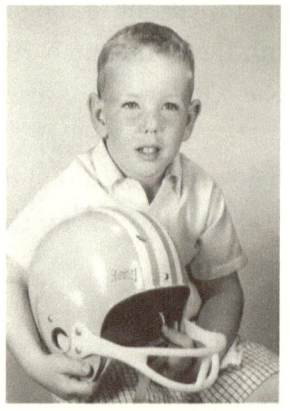

My future is football

Olan Mills Photography

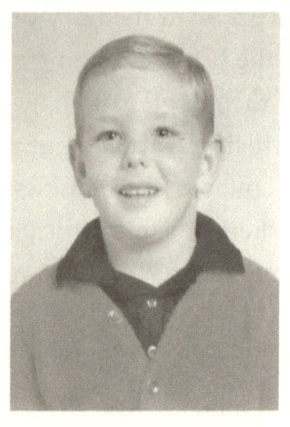

Growing up

East Elementary, Punta
Gorda, Florida

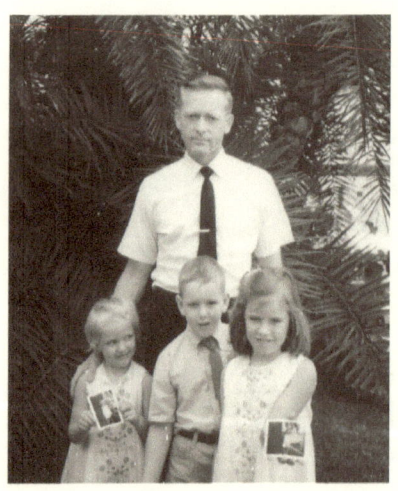

Sunday with Daddy

Mary, Bill, Libby

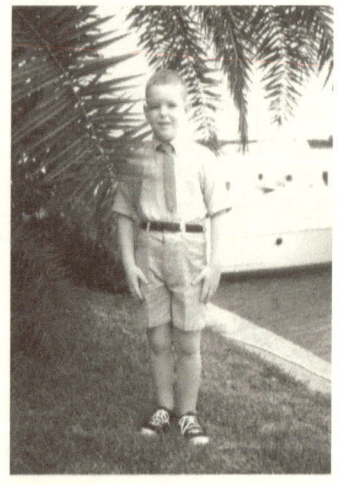

Mama found out I had on
my tennis shoes in church

Vero Beach, Florida

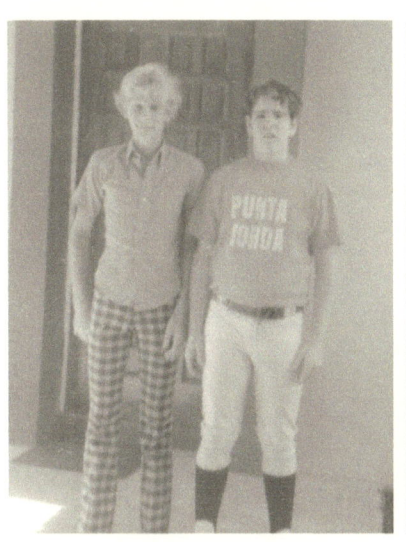
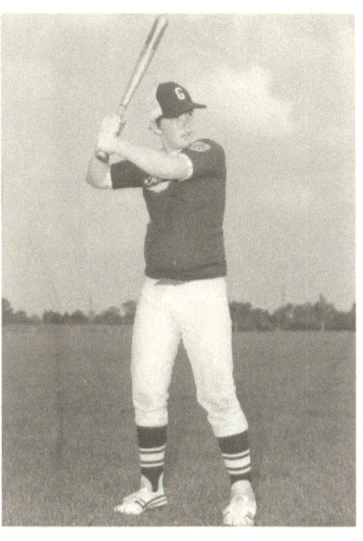

Stephen Parker
and Bill Roddy

It's going over the
fence—pitch it!

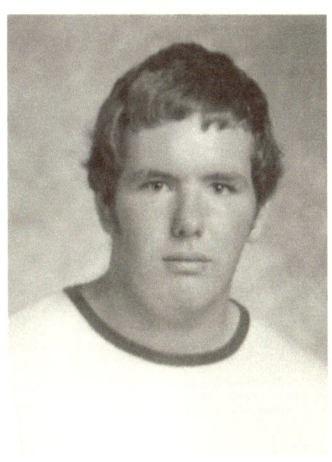

Bill Roddy
Bishop Vero Catholic High
Fort Myers, Florida 1978-1979

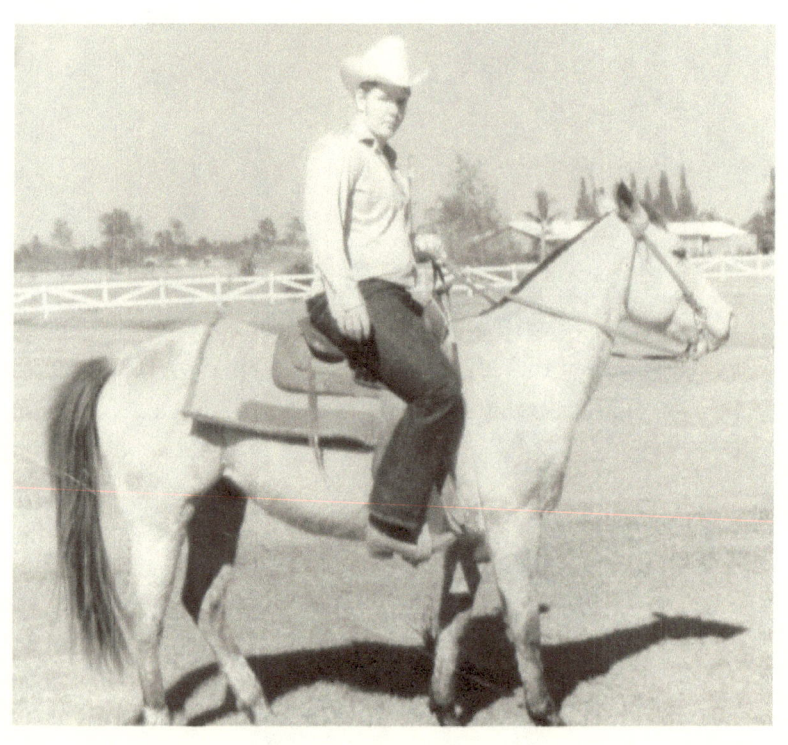

Let's go to Texas
Bill and Shenandoah (Shane)
1979

Chapter Seven
College and Wedding Bells

Libby graduated from SMA and Texas A&M University. After graduation from SMA, Mary and Bill enrolled in Howard Payne University (HPU), a Baptist College in Brownwood, Texas.

Bill shared his life away from home in letters that continued to speak of his love for football, cut short by the shoulder surgery and injuries, and that speak of his faith and God's will.

Dear Mom and Dad,

How is everything going in Seguin? Is the house coming along OK? Everything is going all right up here. I'm having a hard time with the computer class. It has me worried. I wish that you could be up here for the Revival this week. The preacher is really great. I have been going to both services each day. I really don't know what I'm going to do next semester. I don't think that HPU is where I should be. I want to play football again next year and I really don't think I could play up here the way I would like to play. I think about TLC (Texas Lutheran College), but it is not my choice. I have to pray about it and let the Lord tell me the right place where he wants me to be. I don't know how ya'll [sic] feel about my going to TLC? But if I play football next year, which my mind is made up to do, I want to be close to home because it means a lot to me to see you up in the stands. Dad, I know how you feel about my weight and I want to lose it, too, but it is hard to lose weight eating cafeteria food. I hope you can come up one weekend and go to church with us so you can see where we have gone this year. My boss wants to meet you both, and Dad, he was stationed in San Marcos the same time you were in the Army Air Force, I think. I believe ya'll [sic] would really like him. I know that you both think I'm crazy, but my boss has a 1975 Cadillac that looks like it is brand-new, and he wants $2,950.00 for it.

Well, I guess I'll let you go. I have signed up for the computer room from 8 to 10. I'll see you Thanksgiving. I love you.

Love, Bill

We heard a lot about cars from Bill, and he pressured us to get him a vehicle of his own. Bill was fast in almost everything he did, and his father worried about his having an automobile. Often called to the emergency room for surgery on patients involved in automobile accidents, Steve knew firsthand the suffering endured by crash victims. He was not keen on providing wheels for Bill, but finally bought him an old clunker. Bill didn't complain, but his face registered disappointment when he saw his first car. I confronted Steve about the pile of junk parked in the driveway.

"Why did you buy *that* car for Bill?"

"Because the nose is so long, if he's in a wreck, he may survive, and it uses so much gas he can't afford to drive it," he said.

Bill didn't dwell on displeasure with the car his dad bought. He worked at a steel mill all summer and bought a sporty, used Oldsmobile® before he went back to school in the fall.

Although he'd wanted to play football, his shoulders continued to be a problem. He'd met the love of his life at HPU and stayed on at the college in Brownwood.

Steve's health wasn't the best when we had three children in college. Bill's concern is evident in a note he dashed off on his father's stationery:

Dad,

I just want to say bye. I don't know when I'll get back down. You will have to come to Brownwood. We have plenty of room. I hope you get to feeling better. I'll be praying for you. I want to say thank you for everything you have done for me. I don't want you and Mom to worry about Mary. I told Mary I would help her out. I think she might have gotten the job at the mall.

We all love you. We could not have a better dad. If I can do anything for you, let me know.

Love,
Bill

Mary and Caryl Toeppich, an SMA classmate, roomed together at HPU. Mary was not too happy with life in a college dormitory.

"How can I study with the girl next door typing all night and keeping me awake?"

My immediate thought was that the girl who typed also studied. This was the fall of 1982, before computers flooded the market.

From the time the children were toddlers, I prayed someday each would meet and marry a Christian. Bill often joked that I didn't care who he married as long as she was Baptist. Early in 1984, Bill announced his plans to marry the following year on March 9, 1985. When asked, Bill offered pertinent information. "She rooms next door to Mary."

"She isn't the girl who types all night?"

"That's the girl—Carrie Taylor from Austin."

At first, I didn't take Bill seriously, but I should have known better. He planned ahead.

Bill and Carrie married a year later, March 9, 1985. Bill and Carrie's vows in holy matrimony and their years of happy marriage followed the fundamental law of a Christian marriage in God's Word and the teachings of Christ. "For this cause shall a man leave father and mother, and shall cleave to his wife" (Genesis 2:24; Matthew 19:5).

Steve and I were honored by Bill's devotion to Carrie and their children. Over time, we learned that if Bill expressed a goal in words, it became a fact. When Bill and Carrie married, they worked for W. L. Gore & Associates in Austin, Texas, and went to school in the evenings.

Bill called to say they'd bought a mobile home near work, and in four years, they'd buy a house. In four years, as planned, they bought a house in nearby Pflugerville. Their first baby, Christopher, was born the same year—1989. A happy family welcomed baby girl Amanda in 1995.

Bill and Carrie stayed busy at work, with their children's school activities, and their church, First Baptist in Pflugerville, where Carrie worked as director of the Wee Ones program.

★   ★   ★

While our children didn't have trouble cutting the apron strings, I held onto the apron threads. I subjected them to advice on speaking the English language correctly, dressing properly, and using correct manners that I believed necessary for achievement and success in any of their endeavors.

Bill was never a mama's boy; he was his mother's son. Independent and self-sufficient, he would consider motherly advice not necessarily follow it. His entrance into the business world was fodder for continued motherly instruction. My persistent counseling presented opportunities for parody, and Bill's amusement and merriment.

One weekend, I eagerly opened the back door to welcome Bill and Carrie. I was shocked by Bill's appearance. He wore diamond earrings in both ears.

"You can't come into this house until you take those earrings out of your ears," I said.

Bill played up the scene a bit, looked hurt, and then burst out laughing. He slipped off the earrings.

Carrie hastened to explain. "He had me going all over Austin looking for magnetic earrings just so he could see your reaction."

Bill ironed shirts at night to wear to work. During a visit to their home, I watched him iron a dress shirt to wear to a meeting, and I brought up a little corporate protocol.

"At the meeting, remember to pin the name tag on the right side of your coat."

While I was at it, I threw in a morsel on table etiquette, "After finishing your meal, place the silverware with the knife blade turned toward you at the four o'clock position on the plate. This signals the waiter it's okay to remove the plate."

The mothering and less-than-subtle suggestions on etiquette offered prospects for the ridiculous with Bill. If we were eating with others, Bill would catch my eye and, with a twist and flourish of his wrist, place a knife at four o'clock on his plate, sometimes even a paper plate. Then his eyes roved to the left and right to check the plates of others. Discreetly, he signaled the right and wrong placement of silverware on each plate on a table.

Bill thoroughly enjoyed his little charade while I squirmed, fearing he would embarrass guests with, "My mama said—"

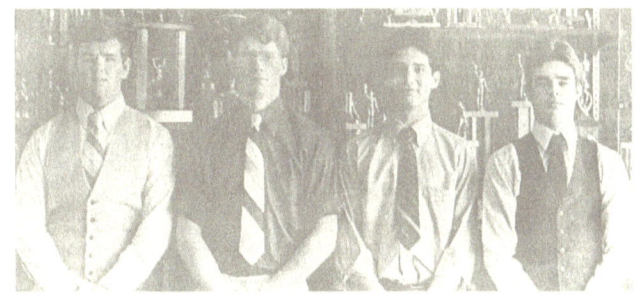

Bill Roddy Scott Stewart Kent Howard Wesley Hollis
San Marcus Baptist Academy
SMA Photo Anders Photography

VARSITY BEARS 1981

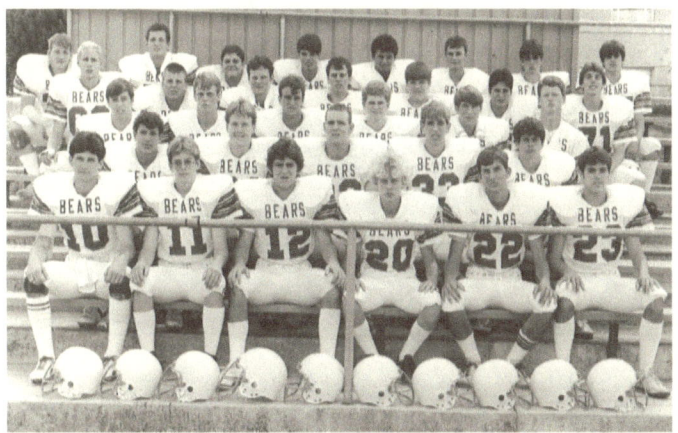

First Row, l-r:K.Howard, D. Spruce, C. Peterson, C. Lee, C. Miertschin, B. Bradford. Second Row, T. Kidd, T. Tannery, B. Roddy, J.D. Hill, R. Duffy. Third Row: T. Lonestar, B. Wiley, A. Davis, S. Stewart. Fourth Row: G. Paluch, T. Dicus, B. Caid, D. Hixson, J. McDowell, W. Vazquez, B. Weldy. Fifth Row: P. Lamb, J. Grimes, J. Francis, B. Dubose, M. Barrios, B. Oliver, J. Rutherford, W. Hollis.

SMA Photos Anders Photography

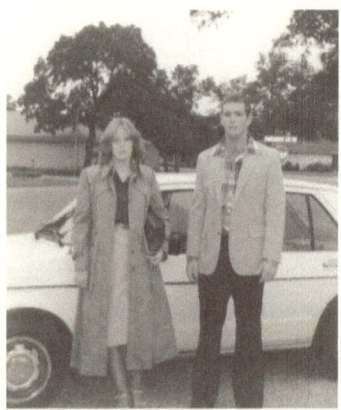 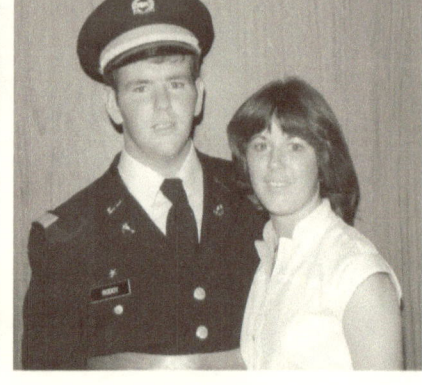

Mary and Bill   Bill and Libby

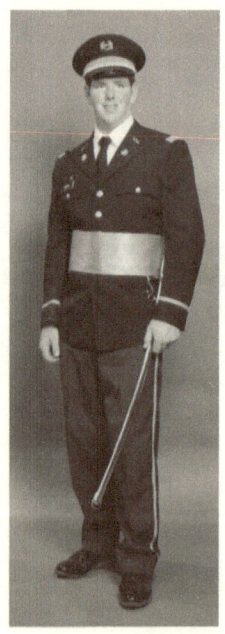

Bill Roddy

Graduation 1981

SMA Photo Anders Photography

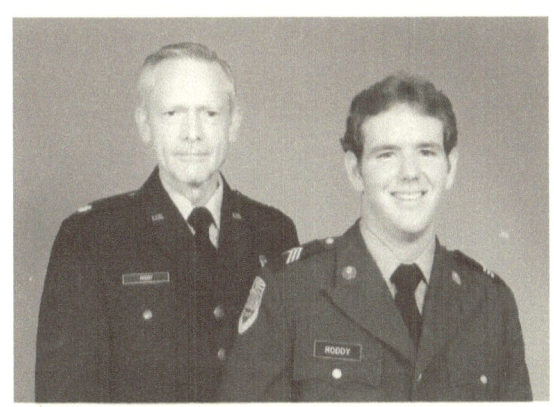

Lt. Col. Stephen R. Roddy, USAFR
SMA ROTC Cadet William Baine Roddy 1981

Photo Courtesy of the Leon Studio Collection of the
Seguin-Guadalupe County Heritage Museum (c)

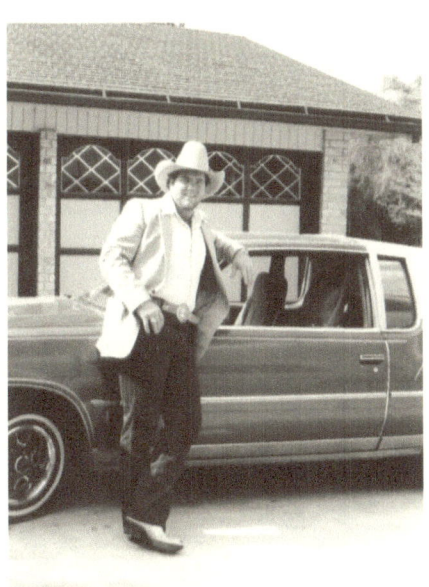

Bill Roddy
Howard Payne University, Brownwood, Texas

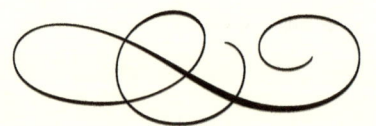

Chapter Eight
Workaday World

I cannot begin to speak about Bill's work history. I was never in a place where he worked. After college and for the next twenty-five years, Bill's work history included three corporations, W. L. Gore & Associates, Dell, Inc., and WORDsearch Corp., producer of Christian e-books to help those who teach and preach. It was gratifying to know our son worked for great and remarkable American companies and worked under men second to none: American businessmen.

Gore manufactures a broad range of products, including waterproof, breathable GORE-TEX® fabrics, implantable medical devices, and wires and cables used in the defense and aerospace industries, among other innovations. Bill worked in their former Austin plant in the cable and cable assembly division. During his time at Gore, Bill traveled to Germany for work. He returned with stories of getting to know fellow associates in the Gore plant and everyday life in Germany. He admired the German people and liked their food, but found the puffy duvets on the beds less than desirable.

On weekends, Bill traveled around Germany. During a snowstorm, an adventurous Bill traveled to Munich with a swing through Switzerland and the Alps. WWII history came alive with Bill's account of Nuremberg's massive stadium during 1938-1939 Nazi party rallies, when young men precision-marched and young women danced across the immense athletic field.

After Gore's Austin plant closed, Bill wrote the CEO a letter thanking him for the work opportunity he and Carrie enjoyed for thirteen years. When they left Gore, a Florida company called Bill for an interview. Bill asked us to babysit Christopher and Amanda in Florida. We met them in the Orlando airport and drove north to a plant on Florida's east coast. We checked into a motel while Bill and Carrie left for interviews. As soon as they were out the door, Steve left the motel for better things to do than babysit. My memory of the day is of being alone in a motel with two little flying missiles. After an exhausting day with his children, I asked Bill about the interview.

He shrugged his shoulders and said, "I can't work for that company. They want to know things about Gore I can't talk about."

When Bill started with Gore, he signed a pledge not to divulge company trade secrets or confidential information, not an uncommon practice in business. It was more than his pledge to Gore that concerned Bill. He had worked for a great company with the highest standards; his mark and word were good. He remained loyal to Gore.

Bill found employment with another company where he worked a few weeks when his boss was transferred. Bill stayed at the company several weeks without the advancement that had been promised earlier.

He applied and was blessed with the opportunity to work for Dell, the world leader in sales of computers, servers, services, and a wide range of products and advanced technology. Bill thrived on the technology and the fast pace of Dell. He was as thrilled and delighted in each new technological advance at Dell as he'd been at Gore. The excitement of pioneering innovations stimulated him. He learned and developed skills at Dell that served him well. He worked at Dell almost ten years until the company was caught up in the slowed economy, which resulted in a major layoff in 2008. Bill could have worked at Dell for a while longer or worked under contract for them, but he made the decision to find another job.

My husband died November 2006. I knew Bill missed his dad. I prayed when Bill left Dell that he'd find employment with an experienced businessman, a mentor, someone with a Judeo-Christian mindset, a good man equal to men and women he'd known at Gore and Dell. It wasn't long before Bill called. He'd interviewed at WORDsearch. If they offered him a job, he planned to take it. My reaction was, "Lord, I prayed for one man. You gave him a whole company."

When WORDsearch hired Bill, little did I know how much the Lord's answer to my prayer and WORDsearch would mean to Bill and to his family.

I can only imagine that Bill's childhood characteristics carried over into his workaday world. His early qualities never seemed to change when he was around me. Bill loved his family and was there for them first. He had an undeniable work ethic, whatever the job.

Bill liked school; he liked work. He was an early riser, and I assumed early to work. He wanted to be first in everything. I wouldn't be surprised to find he was often first at work. He was full of fun and good humor at home and school; he enjoyed his co-workers, he laughed and his fellow workers laughed with him. He made lists for me; he planned ahead on the job.

He didn't like clutter; he was organized. He kept his room clean; he kept his work place clean. Although he'd scoffed at regimentation and protocol, he was disciplined; he believed in a tight rein at work. He could read people and situations; his gift of perception prevailed at work. He was observant and wanted to be on the right page; he was watchful and wanted to get it right at work.

In school and in sports, Bill was where he was supposed to be when he was supposed to be; I presumed the same was true at work. Bill was humble and kind, but could be as bold as a lion. Others saw this trait in him at work.

Chapter Nine
Life in High Gear

By the time he turned forty, Bill and Carrie's lives centered on church, the children's school and sports activities, his work at Dell, and Carrie's work in Wee Ones at First Baptist Church in Pflugerville. They were blessed with children who made professions of faith. They moved from their first house into a larger home in Pflugerville.

In his time off, Bill played as hard as he worked. Sports and NASCAR captured his attention. He delighted in four-wheeler family days on mountain trails in Arkansas. He hunted in Texas and New Mexico, enjoyed boating on Texas lakes, camping, and taking vacations in Florida.

Bill and Carrie remembered us with treasured gifts from their vacations, and mini-dishes with scenes of the Square and the Christmas Market at Nuremberg, Germany, grace our home. A small crystal plaque incised with an image of the bridge at Sydney and an aboriginal figurine came from Australia. Among the thoughtful gifts we received from Bill and Carrie were a beautiful necklace for me and a leather briefcase for Steve from New Zealand; a silver bracelet for me, and a small, black coral sailfish for Steve from Cozumel, Mexico. I'd never heard about black coral, but learned it was a collectible among celebrities. The history and process of making an object interested Bill. He surprised me with his knowledge of crystal, china, and objets d'art not of particular personal interest or value to him. The most meaningful gift from Carrie and Bill was a small copper church that plays "Amazing Grace." I keep the church on the counter above the kitchen sink.

From the year 2000, the lives of our children were on an even keel, except for their father's illnesses when, for six years, Steve was in and out of hospitals. Bill and the girls drove to Houston often to check on us. We looked forward to their visits. They cleaned out the refrigerator, washed clothes, and changed beds. I once found Bill on his knees in the kitchen at five o'clock one morning. He was scrubbing the grout between the floor tiles with a narrow wire brush. My kitchen floor wasn't clean enough to suit him.

In 2005, Bill and Carrie came to Houston on two trips that ultimately involved Hurricanes Katrina and Rita. Bill and Carrie took care of Steve for several days while I met my sister, Ann, and brother, "Brother," in Gloster, Mississippi, to divide furnishings in the house our mother left us. Within weeks, Katrina damaged the house in Mississippi beyond restoration. The next month, advisories filled airwaves on Hurricane Rita spinning in the Gulf of Mexico.

When Bill heard about Rita he said, "Be ready to leave Houston in the morning for Pflugerville, Mom. Rita is headed toward Houston. I want you out of there. With Dad in that hospital bed and all that oxygen equipment, you need to get out."

I protested, but Bill was adamant. "You're leaving tomorrow, Mom. I'm not going to take a chance on your staying in that house."

The next morning, Carrie and her mother, Pat Taylor, arrived with a truck, and we convoyed medical equipment and belongings from Houston to Pflugerville.

Blessed by Bill's intuitive decision, we left Houston ahead of the traffic jams that shut down highways leading out of the city. Although Rita did not cover as wide an area and moved faster than Katrina, it proved to be a major hurricane. Our neighborhood was without electricity for more than a week. We remained with Bill and Carrie in Pflugerville two weeks until the power came back on in our house in Houston.

Through a Dell insurance program for employees, the company provided nursing care for employees' families, including elderly parents. Bill put in a request for a Dell nurse to come to his home during the day while we were in Pflugerville. At night, Bill took over the nursing care of his dad. I'll be forever grateful to Dell, a great company that provided nursing care for one of their employees' bedridden father.

Bill wanted us to move to his neighborhood in Pflugerville so he could help with his dad.

We looked at houses, but I cancelled plans to move to Pflugerville. Bill left for work early in the morning. If I moved to Pflugerville, he would be up most nights with his dad. Taking care of Steve was an around-the-clock effort. I had several nurses in Houston who cared for Steve at home. Demetrica Diamond worked during the day, and Watta Ampadu worked early in the evening and graciously came back anytime of the night when I called.

In 2006, on the day Steve died, the four of us stood by our beloved's bed, held hands, and recited the Twenty-third Psalm.

Bill promised him, "Don't worry, Dad, we'll take care of Mom. Not as good as you did, but we'll take care of her."

Tears rolled down my face. Bill's sincere vow spiced with wit, his own special touch, was typical of our son. I knew if Steve heard Bill, he smiled within his faintly beating heart. It brought back Bill's words to Mary when they were younger. "When Dad's not here, I'm the dad."

Bill was forty-three, and he kept his oath to his father. He stepped up his visits to Houston to check over the house and car. He trimmed the bushes and hedges and cleaned up the yard, faster and better than had been done in years. He went through the house, changing light bulbs to trim my electric bill. He'd give me orders about what to do with this and that. Bill was never more caring than his sisters. They, too, came at every opportunity to help and were always there for me. Bill lived closer to Houston, and it was easier for him to run down for visits.

In 2008, with advisories out on another hurricane in the Gulf and warnings for Houston, Bill called. "Get ready to leave. We're coming for you."

Ike proved to be a major hurricane with homes in the Houston area damaged and a loss of power again for days. I stayed with Bill and Carrie ten days until electricity came back on in my house. Bill and Carrie were well organized and most gracious throughout my long visit. Being with them reminded me of the contrast with my kitchen in disarray—and Steve.

Steve always enjoyed eating with his children and grandchildren at the dining room table. I'd come up with worthy centerpieces and used our good china for the occasions. With fifteen of us, and for more elbow room, we'd set up a cloth-covered card table in the dining room and set the trestle table with china in the breakfast area of our home. Bill protested about the long, drawn-out dinners, leftover food all over kitchen counters, not to mention a sink full of china to hand wash, dry, and put away.

One Christmas, I walked into the dining room to find the centerpiece removed and my good china and crystal replaced with Christmas paper plates and cups and throw-away silver, Bill's idea for a stress-free Christmas Day.

Carrie and Bill's home in Pflugerville was central for the girls and me. They kept their house and kitchen spic-and-span. With Steve gone, they welcomed fourteen of us on several holidays. A buffet of hors d'oeuvres and salads awaited us on their dining table and on kitchen counters, and they served a bounty of warm meats and vegetables from pots on the stove.

Life presented changes. Whether at Carrie and Bill's house or in Greenville at Libby and Jeff's or in Zephyr at Mary and David's, our get-togethers warmed my heart, for the children took great care to preserve our close family fellowship

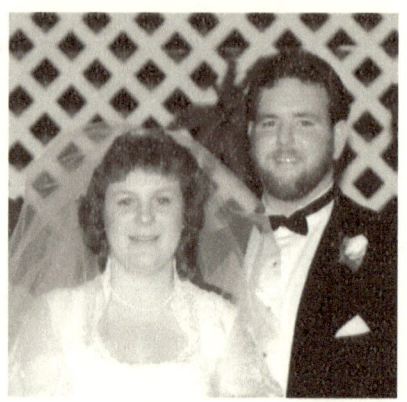

Carrie and Bill
March 1985

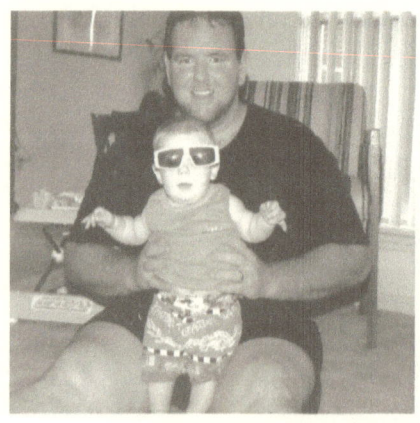

Bill and Christopher
1989

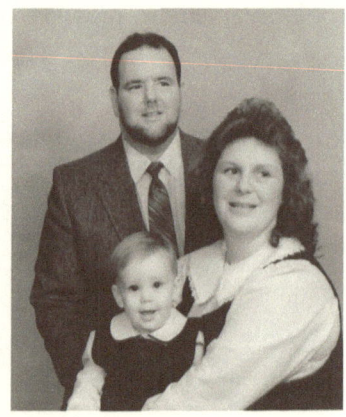

Bill, Carrie, and Christopher
Our first baby 1990

JCPennyStudios/LifeTouch Photo

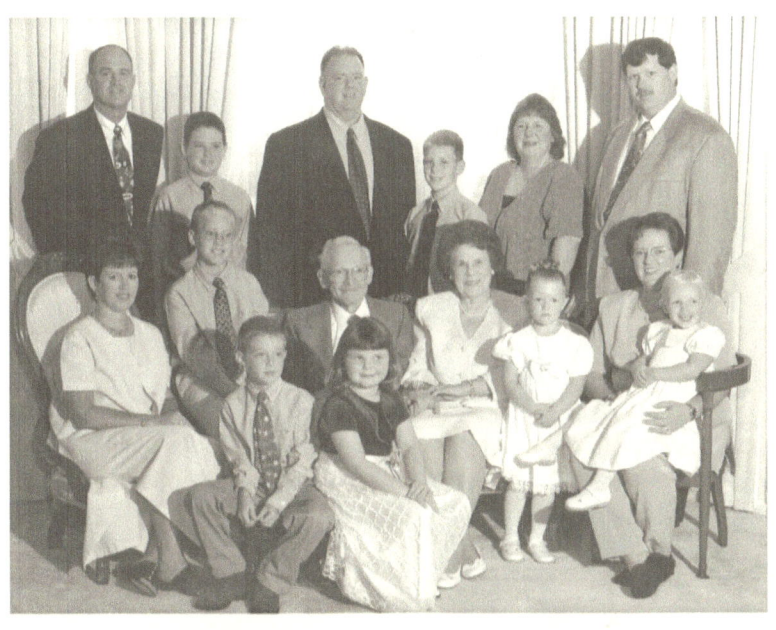

Fiftieth Wedding Anniversary 2001
Back Row: Jeff Rook, Josh Rook, Bill Roddy, Christopher
Roddy, Carrie Roddy, David Howard
Middle Row: Libby Rook, Kyle Rook, Stephen and Martha
Roddy, Samantha Howard, Mary and Andrea Howard
Front Row: Mason Rook and Amanda Roddy

Christine's Photography

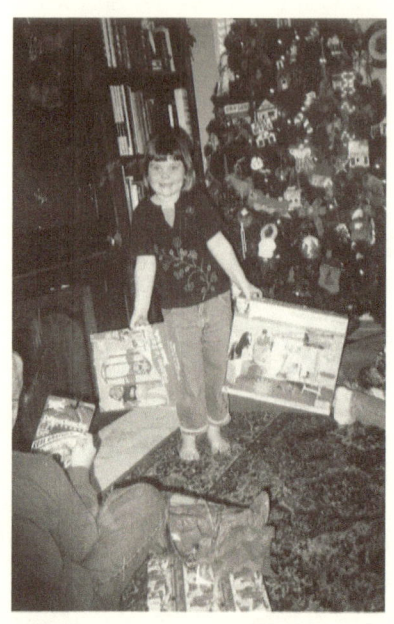

Amanda Roddy
I believe in Daddy!

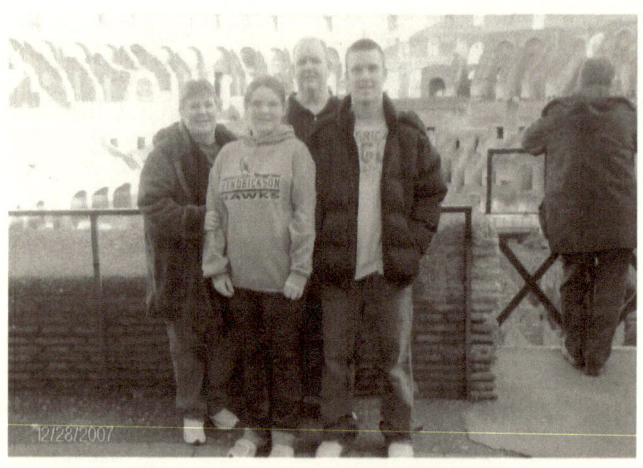

Carrie, Amanda, Bill, Christopher
Coliseum, Rome 2007

Chapter Ten
A Shift in Gears

In April 2009, while in the hospital from the heart attack, Bill was diagnosed with diabetes. He tackled the problem with all his usual fervor and soon had it under control. Doctors signed off for him to return to work within the normal time frame following a stent procedure.

I wasn't surprised but concerned when he called one day during that summer saying he planned to take his children to the Schlitterbahn Waterpark in New Braunfels, Texas. I personally thought he should take it easy in light of the recent heart attack and the fact he had undefined, internal bleeding that had required six units of blood to get him up, out, and about. It became clear to me that he had no intention of taking life easy or canceling the long Fourth of July family weekend in Florida he'd planned months earlier.

In August 2009, there was evidence for the first time that the source of Bill's bleeding was the colon, and a colonoscopy revealed a large mass in the upper right colon. Physicians recommended surgery as soon as possible, but Bill didn't cotton for one second to the idea of being inconvenienced by surgery.

Before his surgery, Bill wanted Christopher settled at Tabor College, a Mennonite college, in Hillsboro, Kansas, where he had signed to play football. In early September, Bill and Carrie went with Christopher to enter for the fall semester. When they told their son about the tumor, Tabor football coaches rallied around Christopher and became prayer warriors for Bill and the family.

Several of us closest to Bill encouraged him to seek the best hospital and doctor for surgery, and we were prepared to give it our all to see that he received the best treatment possible.

I thought of my husband and missed him and the health advice that I'd considered second to none. The privileged counsel we had experienced for years was over. Bill had a critical health decision to make on his own—with one exception—his faith in God.

At his best on a computer, Bill researched the Internet for top hospitals and surgeons to consider. He was aware of what was going on in the treatment and surgery arena of colon cancer surgery. He quoted statistics for survival and deliberated his options with his usual strength and energy. He decided by whom, when, and where he'd have the surgery.

Focusing on hospitals and doctors with the highest survival rates to conquer his enemy, cancer, he seriously considered Mayo Clinic in Rochester, Minnesota, or Mayo's in Jacksonville, Florida, and M. D. Anderson Cancer Center in Houston. My father, brother, and husband had been through Mayo Clinic in Rochester, and I felt comfortable with Mayo's for Bill. At M. D. Anderson Cancer Center in Houston, I had received the best treatment under the care of Patrick M. Lynch, M.D., gastroenterologist, who had successfully removed the large precancerous polyp.

Bill weighed the line of scrimmage to win the game of life and began transferring medical records to M. D. Anderson.

Chapter Eleven
A Bump in the Road

Bill and Carrie lived in Pflugerville, and Bill worked in Austin. There were several holdups transferring medical records from Austin to M. D. Anderson and scheduling an appointment at the famed cancer center. In the interim, Bill searched nearer home and work for surgeons to review his case.

In Austin, he found that with laparoscopic surgery, recovery time was shorter than with a midline incision. Except for routine pre-surgery tests, there was no delay scheduling surgery in Austin. Bill wanted the tumor out, so he chose Austin where he could get on the surgery schedule quickly for the *modus operandi*, laparoscopic removal of the tumor, the procedure with the shortest recovery time. Also, he factored in that he'd be closer to home and work during recovery and recuperation.

Surgery for removal of the colon mass was performed the third week in September in Austin. Laboratory reports confirmed a malignant tumor. Out of seventeen lymph nodes removed, eleven were malignant with no evidence of metastases found in major organs. The tumor was classified stage III, within a curable percentage range for survival—a paradox.

Recovery from surgery was uneventful, and Bill felt better each day. After his discharge from the hospital, Carrie went back to work. I stayed with them a week, hoping to be of help to Bill. He was up and around and out of the house in a few days. Before being released by doctors to go back to work, he was off to Kansas on weekends to watch Christopher play football. Some weekends, he'd fly, and other weekends he'd drive with Carrie and Amanda.

A thank you note came from Bill after my return to Houston. The envelope was postmarked October 5, 2009.

Mom,

Thank you so much for all you did for me. Thank you also for all the prayers. This is just a bump in the road, and I'll be OK. Look forward to KC.

Love you,
Bill

While he was recuperating from surgery, and before he had a medical release to go back to work, Bill asked me to join them for two football trips. He looked good and never complained on either trip.

In late October, we drove to Hillsboro for homecoming weekend at Tabor College. Hillsboro had one motel, and Bill made reservations at a bed and breakfast. I couldn't help but laugh when the hostess served a nice breakfast on her best china with crystal goblets, not exactly Bill's idea of a football weekend. After we left the charming bed and breakfast, Bill remarked he'd never go back to another bed and breakfast; he'd rather eat at Denny's.

On the second trip, I went with them for a football game near Kansas City. Bill reserved motel rooms in Kansas City, Missouri, where I grew up. We spent one morning driving around my old neighborhood. After more than sixty-six years, I was thrilled to see where I had lived and my old elementary school, Faxon, on Paseo Boulevard. We parked at First Baptist Church (now Metropolitan Baptist) on Linwood, where I attended Sunday school, vacation Bible school, and was baptized. The words *First Baptist* engraved in stone over the main entrance of my old church caught my eye. I wanted to walk through the doors and see the sanctuary once again.

"Mom, there's a hearse and hundreds of cars in this parking lot," Bill said. "A big funeral is going on at the church. Someone important died. We can't go in that sanctuary."

I was so excited to see my church that I hadn't even noticed the hearse or the cars.

We left and visited the Plaza, a site of happy memories, and Nelson-Atkins Art Gallery, where I'd attended Saturday art classes. In Union Station, we stood under the clock I well remembered. We toured Truman Library in Independence, Missouri. We found President Truman and the First Lady's garments hung from pegs in the museum. Bill donned a flowered shirt worn by President Truman in Key West, and Amanda slipped into a blouse belonging to First Lady Bess Truman. We treasure hilarious photographs of Bill and Amanda dressed in President Truman and the First Lady's clothes.

On the Kansas City trip, we toured the Missouri and Kansas countryside along the Missouri River. We drove by the well-known federal prison and through the grounds of the military hospital in Leavenworth, Kansas, and the impressive Leavenworth National Cemetery.

Bill remarked about the beauty of the white crosses covering the hilly terrain of the national cemetery and its perpetual care. He stopped the car to read dates on markers on the graves of veterans. In another sobering moment, Bill reflected on graves of men, younger than he, who gave their lives for our country. With our American flag waving over row after row of crosses, sentinels of allegiance to "one nation under God, indivisible, with liberty and justice for all," freedom rang out loud and clear. The visit to the Leavenworth National Cemetery stirred our hearts.

Our sightseeing included Amelia Earhart Birthplace Museum in Atchison, Kansas, a site that offers motivation for young women and men pursuing careers in aviation.

On our tours throughout the weekend, we empathized with great Americans who lived and died nobly for causes dear to their hearts. The sites we visited would inspire anyone with confidence and hope. Bill was positive and upbeat throughout the weekend, and we were filled with optimism for his future.

Bill wrote as he spoke, concisely. I suggested keeping a journal of his experience with cancer to write a book later.

"Why would I want to write about it?"

I didn't press the issue, but Bill did write about cancer. Throughout his battle, he kept a laptop by his side. He communicated with friends, and every line he read on the social media encouraged him.

"You won't believe who I heard from today, a girl from first grade at East."

I wasn't into social networking. Julia Todd, my friend and neighbor, invited me over to read multiple postings to and from Bill on her computer. He shared his encounter with the "Big C" with friends and family, giving updates, spreading hope and comfort. Tears rolled down my face when I read the Bible verses he posted and his banner, "It's in the Lord's hands; I'm just along for the ride."

Bill didn't wait until later to share his experience with cancer. He opened his heart to others, and they opened their hearts to him. He expressed his trust and faith in his Savior to the world on the Internet, and an army of prayer warriors from all over supported him.

Pen strokes on paper, strikes on a computer keyboard are worthless unless they circuit into the hearts of others. Bill connected.

In November 2009, Bill went back to work about the time the chemotherapy began, which he tolerated with few side effects. In December, something near his right lung showed up on a CAT scan. The oncologist opted to watch the area and continue the same treatment. In January 2010, Bill's doctors advised he was doing well, and if he continued, he'd be off chemo in April and on the five-year routine follow-up regime. Our hopes were high.

In February 2010, WORDsearch moved Bill to the sales call center. He was thrilled and excited with the new challenge. In 2002, he had sold AdvoCare® at night and on weekends and won a ten-day luxury trip for two to Australia and New Zealand. He knew he could sell, and I did too. Bill had the giddy-up-and-go. He was a born salesman. His life was back on track again.

February 14, 2010, brought delight and laughter with a package from Bill. My Valentine's present was a large, red, heart-shaped box of chocolates topped with an enormous sack of orange slices, my favorite candy.

Later in February, a CAT scan showed the colon cancer had metastasized in both Bill's lungs. In March, undaunted with the latest report, Bill and Carrie flew to San Francisco, as planned, for their twenty-fifth wedding anniversary. They had a wonderful time touring the area and climbing the hills of San Francisco. The highlight of their trip was visiting with Leslie Brandon Ackerman, a lifelong family friend, from Punta Gorda, Florida, now married and living in California. Libby and Leslie's birthdays are a day apart. Bill had long since forgiven and forgotten that Leslie joined Libby in calling him Baby Bill. Although it took him awhile to forgive, he never forgot another incident involving Libby and Leslie.

His obsession with NASCAR began one Christmas with a go-kart under the tree. To Bill's dismay, Libby and Leslie slyly raced off in his treasured vehicle. He was surprised to hear the go-kart motor start up, and he ran out the back door and found the two Ls spinning around the backyard in his go-kart. I'll never forget the scene.

Bill jumped up and down and his face showed utter and complete anguish, "What are they doing? They are going to wreck my go-kart! They are going to hit that ditch. They don't know what they're doing. Come back here! Just look at them—they're laughing! They're tearing up my go-kart. Oh, look what they've done! They've ruined my go-kart!"

I don't remember the go-kart being harmed. Through the years, though, the mere mention of the escapade never failed to bring laughter to the Brandon and Roddy families.

Bill and Carrie returned from San Francisco and went back to their jobs. Bill resumed riding his bike late in the afternoons. I received a gift package with a can of clam chowder, a sourdough bread bowl, and chopsticks that they had shipped from California.

On March 23, 2010, we learned that Kitsy Campbell, Bill's cousin, died unexpectedly. Kitsy's personality was similar to Bill's, outgoing with a sense of humor, a real people person. She loved getting together with family as much as Bill. Both enjoyed cooking. A connoisseur of food, Kitsy delighted in sharing epicurean dinners with the family she loved. Bill and Kitsy were close and kept in touch. She'd visited Bill and Carrie in Texas several times.

The same day Kitsy died, Bill experienced a moment of spiritual significance while driving home from work. "I heard an inner voice say, 'I will take care of you.'" Bill shared this experience with me the last time I was alone with him, on April 17, 2010.

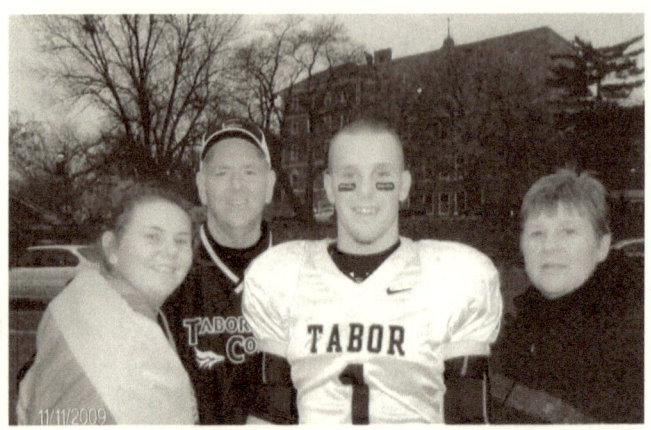

Amanda, Bill, Christopher, Carrie
Tabor College 2009

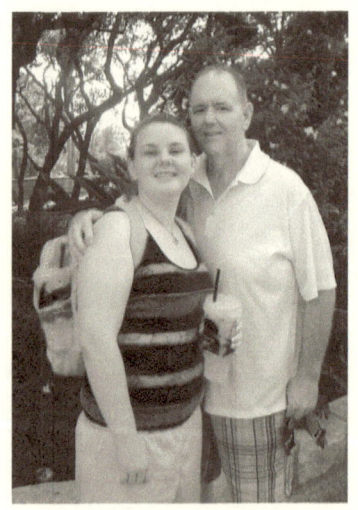

Amanda and Bill
San Antonio, Texas 2009

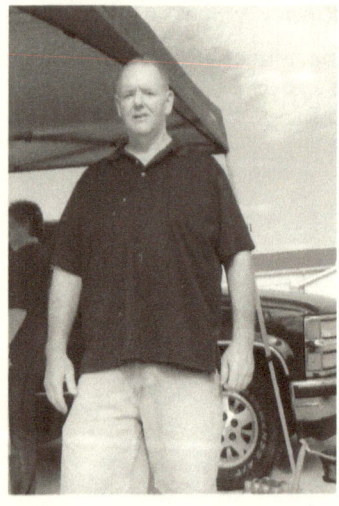

Bill Roddy
Tailgating at Tabor College
2009

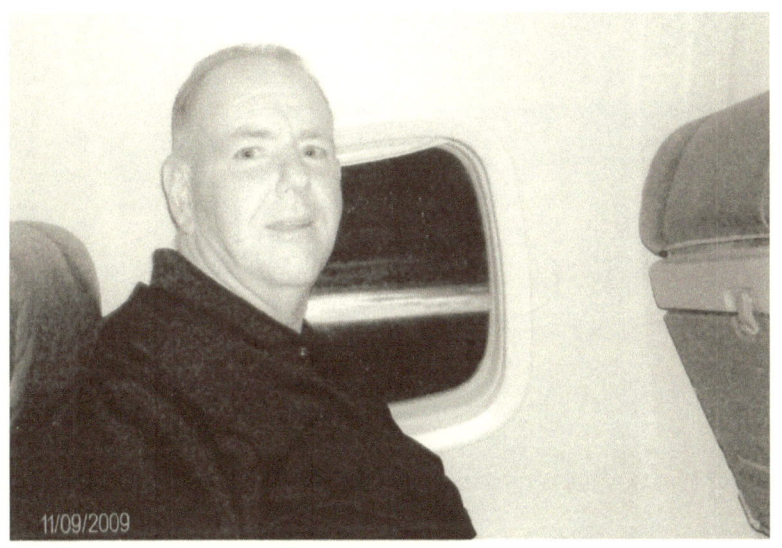

William Baine Roddy
Just along for the ride
Flight to Kansas City, Missouri

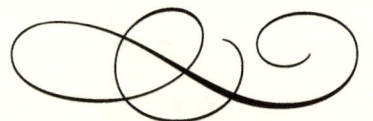

Chapter Twelve
The Override

On March 24, 2010, Bill went to M. D. Anderson, Houston, for the first time since he'd been diagnosed with colon cancer, for a second opinion on the latest report showing metastases to his lungs. He rushed through the long corridors at MDA with Carrie and his friend, Delonda Delony, an RN and former classmate at San Marcos Academy. I puffed to keep up with them.

Three days later, on Easter Sunday, Bill was hospitalized in Austin with pneumonia. We presented Bill with an Easter basket filled with fun, including a plastic worm. Bill hung the realistic, gross worm on the IV rack. Normally calm nurses jumped back in fright when they reached up to change IVs, much to Bill's amusement and our laughter.

Bill was hospitalized in Austin until a few days before his next appointment at MDA on April 9, 2010. When he returned to the hospital for the second appointment and consideration in clinical trials, physicians admitted him to the hospital.

Mary, David, and their girls, Samantha and Andrea, visited Bill that first weekend at M. D. Anderson. Bill laughed and joked with his nieces. He didn't look sick. The following week, Paul Petropolis drove to the hospital and met Bill. His visit was special to Bill. Paul, a sports writer and cancer survivor himself, founded Angels in Action, the organization that ministers to cancer victims and their families in Houston and other cities.

On Saturday, April 17, Bill and his lifelong friend, Stephen Parker, planned to take in the NASCAR race in Fort Worth. With Bill still in M. D. Anderson, Stephen deplaned in Houston from his flight to Fort Worth and the NASCAR event.

My neighbors knew Bill was in the hospital in Houston and brought food to the house for the family. I mentioned the great food available at home. A celebration was at hand for Bill.

"Hey, Mom, bring those chickens, that potato salad, cookies, all that food down here. We'll have a picnic in my room and watch NASCAR," he said.

Stephen and I packed up the food at the house for the get-together. We had the picnic, although the NASCAR race was rained out that Saturday in Fort Worth. Bill announced during the afternoon that he had tickets for his family of four to attend the NASCAR event in Bristol, Virginia, in August 2010.

Later on that Saturday, Jeff and Libby arrived to be with Bill. We pushed him in a wheelchair with the IV rack attached to the indoor park at the hospital. Surrounded by his family and a friend, Bill laughed and joked with us about good times. He said he felt good. He was happy, especially since Christopher and his baby girl, Amanda, who turned fifteen in February, came from Pflugerville to be with him.

The family group left for dinner, and I stayed with Bill in his room. Bill didn't feel as well as he had earlier in the day. He had a few issues on his mind. He'd requested a physical therapist to walk him to keep his strength up. The hospital sent an occupational therapist who suggested Bill write letters to his wife and children.

"He tells me I'm dying with cancer, and I have time to write letters to my wife and my children to tell them I love them. I don't need to write letters to them. They know I love them. They're struggling with this more than I am."

To keep his strength up, he asked me to arrange for Jeff Rook, Libby's husband, and Stephen Parker, his Florida friend, to walk with him.

"I don't need their help," he said. "I want them to push a wheelchair behind me."

From the beginning, I believed, and still believe, that God can heal instantly. I prayed for God's grace and glory in the course of Bill's struggle with cancer. I believed in the fifth commandment, "Honor thy father and mother, that long life may be on the land which the Lord thy God giveth thee" (Exodus 20:12). Bill was wonderful to us. I clung to the promise that Bill, in honoring his parents, secured long life, a reward for his love and respect for Steve and me. I prayed in God's will; in my heart, I believed the Lord would heal my son. I needed him. More than that, Carrie, Christopher, and his baby girl Amanda needed him.

I knew his situation was critical. I prayed for a miracle, believing the Lord wouldn't take him. God was the ultimate caregiver. I'd never given up credence that Bill would be healed instantly and survive. "'For my thoughts are not your thoughts, neither are your ways my ways, saith the Lord. 'For as the heavens are higher than the earth, so are my ways, and my thoughts from your thoughts'" (Isaiah 55:8-9).

Bill's insight into the feelings of others rarely failed him. He had an issue, not about God's instant healing, but with me. He brought up the subject when the family left for dinner and the two of us were alone. Bill promised his dad he'd take care of me, and on this last time we were alone, he brought up the issue of God's will for him, my beloved son. He shared the powerful proclamation he heard on March 23.

"I believe the Lord can heal instantly. He can heal twenty-two patients tonight or three patients tonight, with what I have. I believe it. I want to believe it. On March 23, driving home from work, I heard a voice that said, 'I will take care of you.' God will take care of me."

Bill knew God healed instantly. He wanted to be on the exact page with God, the right page this Saturday night. His life was in God's hands and will. It was crucial to him that his mother was on the right page—the exact page with God too. He wanted me to let go and be in God's will and accept what God willed for him. He'd promised his dad he'd take care of me. Being assured that I was in God's will was taking care of me and an issue for him.

We both teared up. I told Bill I loved him, and he told me he loved me. With our arms around each other, I prayed for Bill's healing—in God's will. Bill and I were on the same page.

About that time, the family walked through the door. Bill sniffed a brief moment, and then asked, "What's up?"

Someone asked if he was okay. He assured them that everything was okay.

Bill told me that night what he'd been telling everyone all along, "It's in the Lord's hands. I'm just along for the ride."

I came home from the hospital and searched for comfort in the Bible. I found the Scripture about Jesus healing ten lepers at once, and only one turned back, "and with a loud voice glorified God" (Luke 17:11-19, author's paraphrase).

I had prayed in God's will for His grace and glory in Bill's fight with cancer. My thoughts centered on Bill winning the battle over cancer and *living*. I couldn't imagine life on Earth without Bill or any one of my children or grandchildren. I prayed with all my heart for God's will not mine, but never let go of Bill surviving the cancer.

Satan wears many hats. He has the ability to distract us from life's problems and pressures. Unfortunately, he has the power to invade our innermost thoughts and feelings and our actions. Satan pounced on my vulnerability in prayers for Bill, in my choice and not God's will, of my son's life span. Satan, the ultimate deceiver and manipulator was subtle with me. Adept at disguises, the most notorious intelligence agents pale in comparison to Satan's undercover attire. Satan attempted to mimic God when I was on my knees in prayer. Bill looked into my heart, recognized a twist within the depths of my soul, and confronted me about being in God's will all the way.

Bill was on track. Twenty-two patients or three patients could be healed in God's will that night. It was essential to pray in God's will. God saves armies in his mighty power. Bill believed in instant healing. He believed in the override—God's will—more.

In the *San Marcos Daily Record* on Sunday, October 4, 1981, Russell Smith, sports editor, wrote that Bill wasn't embittered with the losing 1981 San Marcos Academy football team.

Bill's outlook on the circumstances of life never changed. He never expressed bitterness in his struggle with cancer. He comforted and led others in God's will. His mission in life seemed to be taking care of others. One of his last duties on Earth was to take care of his mother and correct her course, in God's will.

God's promises are not based on rewards for works. God promises eternal life. In his valiant struggle with cancer, Bill's faith in God's will glorified God's magnificence and power. "For God so loved the world, he gave his only begotten Son, that whosoever believeth in him should not perish, but have everlasting life" (John 3:16).

The Lord gave me forty-six years of a bundle of joy. Bill knew God would take care of him. Time after time, the Lord protected our children. I recalled a day the Lord kept Steve and Bill from harm.

The summer before we left Florida, I'd never heard of Frank Merriwell, but Steve witnessed his son in a Frank Merriwell moment. Bill attended a youth retreat at Stetson University in Deland, Florida. A key speaker at the event was Bobby Bowden, famed football coach of the Florida State University. Bill admired Bobby Bowden as much as he did Bear Bryant, the University of Alabama coach. Football season offered an opportunity for Steve to take Bill to see Bobby Bowden in action at an FSU game in Tallahassee. The two of them left Punta Gorda on a small, two-engine plane that serviced Charlotte County Airport in Punta Gorda and smaller Florida airports.

At home, I felt uneasy when Steve and Bill were late coming in from the Tallahassee ball game. I walked outside and could not find a dark cloud in the sky. I knew the weather wasn't holding them up. I alternated between looking at the clock and peeking out the front door at Highway 74 for a glimpse of Steve's car.

When I saw Steve's Datsun 280Z® turn into our country subdivision, I breathed a sigh of relief and ran to the carport to give hugs. They both looked and acted a little strange.

"Why are you all so late getting here?"

"Getting here? I didn't think we'd make it back," Steve said.

On the return trip from Tallahassee, less than fifty miles from Punta Gorda and near the Sarasota Airport, things went awry with the plane's electrical system. The plane's lights and the radio went out. One motor failed. The pilot decided to land at the smaller airport in Punta Gorda, which was forty miles farther away. Bill sat opposite the pilot in the front, while Steve sat in one of the backseats next to a lady who could not speak English. Understandably, she became unglued at their plight. On the approach to the Charlotte County Airport, the pilot struggled to get the landing gear down. It wouldn't budge. Facing a crash on the runway, the pilot asked Bill to try to dislodge the landing gear. With tremendous effort, Bill moved the landing gear extension and lowered the plane's wheels moments before the plane touched down.

Steve's brisk account of the last fifty miles of their flight sent shivers through my body. I empathized with the terrified lady who clung to him. Then I asked Steve what he did to calm his fellow passenger.

"In her hysterical state, she couldn't respond to anything. She had me in a death grip. If it hadn't been for Bill, we wouldn't be here." Steve spoke in awe of Bill's calm demeanor. "Our boy saved four lives."

Bill seemed unusually quiet. I asked what he was thinking during their ordeal.

"Kicking the door out and jumping when the plane got closer to the ground."

How thankful we were for God's care on that particular day. There were other times God protected Bill. I remembered the night a herd of cattle broke loose on the highway not far from our house near Punta Gorda. Bill jumped on a horse and raced off to help with the roundup. In Steve's car, we chased after Bill, fearing he would be hurt. Steve slammed on the car brakes when we saw the horse sans rider standing by the highway. We lowered the windows and heard Bill moaning in the roadside ditch. The saddle had slipped, and he'd fallen from the racing horse. On another occasion, Bill had a car wreck in San Marcos. He received slight concussions from both accidents, and it was difficult keeping him quiet. Then, less than a year ago, during his heart attack, Bill staggered into an emergency room in Austin. Quick-thinking medical personnel and doctors saved his life.

I looked back with gratitude for God's astounding care through the years. The Lord had given us days of precious moments with our beloved son and given him many days to inspire others with his witness in God's will. I knew God was there for Bill and all of us on this day at M. D. Anderson.

In the Bible, Mary and Martha sent for Jesus when their brother, Lazarus, became ill.

"When Jesus heard that, he said, 'This sickness is not unto death, but for the glory of God, that the Son of God might be glorified thereby'" (John 11:4).

Chapter Thirteen
In His Grace and Glory

Sunday, April 18, the family and Stephen Parker, his lifelong friend, were back in Bill's room in the hospital.

Before he left for Florida, Stephen Parker put his hand on Bill's shoulder. "Take care, brother," he said. They were truly brothers, as Scripture says, "A man that hath friends, must show himself friendly: and there is a friend that sticketh closer than a brother" (Proverbs 18:24). Touched by the depth of their friendship, I walked out of the room with Stephen and a nurse.

I said to the nurse, "These two guys are wonderful men."

Stephen winked at the nurse and grinned. "She doesn't know everything."

With a mother's instinct, my thought was, *I do know everything. You were the friskiest boys in the world, now you're the best of the best men in the world. Committed to the Lord, devoted family men, hard workers, patriotic Americans to the core, you honor your families and your parents and never whine. You are steadfast, charitable Christian men.*

Bill's friends were prototypes of Stephen, brothers and sisters cut from the same cloth, fine upstanding men and women at church and work and in their communities.

Libby and Mary, God's girls and their brother's soul mates, were at his side in the hospitals and in prayer throughout his struggle with cancer. Friends from San Marcos Baptist Academy and unwavering Christians and friends of all faiths stood by Bill, including Mike Draper, SMA and NASCAR buddy, who visited often with Bill. Jeff Price and Bobby Plyler, Delonda Delony, and other SMA friends came to see Bill while I was in his room. Friends came from Gore, Dell, and WORDsearch to support Bill. He appreciated each of them. Udo Hafner, another NASCAR pal, worked with Bill at Gore, Dell, and WORDsearch. Udo came to walk with Bill in the hospital following the colon surgery. David Howard and Jeff Rook, his brothers-in-law, were there for him. His pastors, Reverends Steve Washburn and John Woods, supported him in prayer and friendship. Church friends sustained Bill and his family with food and constant prayer.

Bill's friends were the backbone of America, God's men and women. One of their own was down, and they rallied around him in never-to-be-forgotten love, and he gave back to them in the grace and glory of God.

Stephen's mother, Gale Parker, said that Stephen thought Bill looked tired when he visited him in Houston. He *was* getting tired.

On Monday, April 19, Bill asked to be taken off pain medication because it made him too drowsy. He wanted to be alert so he could know what was going on. A specialist at the hospital checked Bill for an infection in the lungs. Later, the infectious disease physician came into the room to report that there was no infection, and that Bill's stats were better. The same day, other doctors came in to tell Bill he wasn't a candidate for clinical trials, and that cancer was taking over his lungs. While Bill tried smoking in college, he wasn't a smoker. He complained cigarette smoke made him sick, and he even campaigned against smoking. Still, cancer cells were devouring his healthy lungs.

Bill had a plan. He thought research hospitals received different drugs in clinical trials. If only he could get stronger, he'd try for acceptance in a clinical trials unit at the University of Texas in San Antonio. We gathered medical records most of the day on Monday, April 19. I planned to drive to San Antonio the next day to hand-deliver the records, but Bill overheard the discussion between Carrie and me about my driving to San Antonio. "Don't do that," he said. "Fax those records."

The clinical trials unit in San Antonio agreed. I faxed ninety pages of medical records to San Antonio that Monday.

Carrie remained at Bill's bedside night and day, taking care of his every need while he was in the hospital in Austin, as well as at M. D. Anderson. Her care and love for Bill never ceased, day after day. On Tuesday, April 20, Bill was awake most of the day and able to get out of bed, but he was weaker.

I took a favorite of his, an oven-roasted turkey sandwich, to him, hoping that eating would help keep up his strength. He didn't eat the sandwich, but later ate from a dinner tray Carrie ordered for him.

Carrie called Wednesday morning, saying that MDA might discharge Bill to a palliative care unit in Austin. She called again to say that the ambulance to transfer Bill would be there at 2:30 that afternoon. I tried, but didn't have time to get to the hospital before Bill and Carrie left for Austin. I suppressed an urge to park on the feeder at US 290 nearby and wave when the ambulance passed on the way to Austin.

Delonda Delony stayed with Bill and Carrie at the hospital in Houston. She noticed that the oxygen mask made it difficult for Bill to talk, as he gave the ambulance attendant the okay sign with his thumb and forefinger. He was still very alert. There was a delay at the parking ramp on that scorching hot day. Delonda observed Bill's irritation in the ambulance that felt like an oven in the mid-afternoon heat. She stayed with Bill and Carrie until the ambulance left M. D. Anderson at 3:30 in the afternoon, and then drove to my house to bring their luggage from the hospital.

We planned to drive Bill's dark red Ford® sedan, parked in my driveway, to Pflugerville on Thursday, and Delonda loaded Bill's car with luggage and oxygen equipment brought from Austin.

Sometime after seven o'clock, Delonda and I heard from Carrie. Bill had made the trip to Austin and said, "Good," when they arrived. About thirty minutes after their arrival, Carrie called to tell me to come to Austin. After receiving a shot, Bill's breathing had become worse. Doctors told Carrie Bill wouldn't make it through the night.

Delonda went into action. "Get your things. I'm driving you to Austin right now."

She loaded everything from Bill's car into her truck. Several neighbors gathered in the drive as we left for Austin. I called Libby and Mary from Delonda's truck.

"What happened?" Libby asked.

I knew the last time Libby saw Bill three days before, he didn't seem to have so little time. I looked at my watch. It was 8:15. The sun was setting.

Carrie called my cell to find out where we were on our way to Austin. We'd just passed Bastrop less than twenty miles away. Within minutes to Bill's bedside, we passed the Austin-Bergstrom Airport. An airliner flew low over the highway. Bill's enthusiasm for travel crossed my mind. A pilot was in full control of the plane; God was in full control of Bill.

"Hey, Mom, I'm okay. I'm on my way. I'm in the Lord's hands. I'm just along for the ride."

I knew that Bill was heaven-bound.

The Lord took Bill home the very day he left M. D. Anderson, Wednesday, April 21, 2010, at 10:37 pm. Delonda and I arrived at the palliative care facility five minutes later. I walked into the room. My son's skin was still warm and moist to my touch. Mary and David arrived within the next ten minutes. Libby was on her way from Waco. Bill's pastor, Reverend Steve Washburn, called Jeff in Greenville to divert Libby from the palliative care unit in Austin to the house in Pflugerville.

We left Austin for Bill and Carrie's house. My heart ached in sorrow for my son and anguished over his sister driving alone on the highway. It seemed to take Libby a long time to drive from Waco to Pflugerville. A weight lifted from my heart when I heard her enter the house. She fell into my and Mary's arms. Together, we shared our sorrow for our beloved son and brother. We knew Bill was with the Lord. He was where he was supposed to be.

Always ready to go and the first to be there, Bill was the first of our precious children to leave for his heavenly home.

This unedited poem, found after his death, reminds me of April 21, 2010.

The Greatest Defeat
by
Bill Roddy

Harvey Haddix, Pittsburgh Pirate,
went out to play
in 1959 on a warm 29th
of May.

At the end of the nine innings
not a single Milwaukee had improved
their slim livings,
and now had one foot in the grave.

The Pirates had been on base several times
but no one scored against the Braves.

And the whole game was
tied up in a net.
Extra innings were played
tenth, eleventh, and twelfth.

Haddix's perfect game ended as
a farce;
Montilla rounded third and
came in with a winning run.

But Aaron who thought the ball was
inside the park,

headed accidentally for the dugout
And the game was won
not by the Pirates
but by the Milwaukee Braves.

The cancer didn't win. The cancer was a farce. Bill was in the Lord's care. Bill's home-going was colon cancer's greatest defeat. He was down in the last inning and hit a home run all the way to heaven. Steady, he landed on his feet and began life everlasting.

Bill Roddy was a people person and people will remember his warmth and laughter, and most of all his devotion to his Savior. Bill hit the ball out of the park on April 21, 2010, and in his passing, he glorified God.

★   ★   ★

On April 24, 2010, the Saturday after our picnic at M. D. Anderson, our family gathered with Carrie, Christopher, and Amanda in Pflugerville to commemorate Bill's life. With aching hearts, my daughters and their children stood with me. Kyle, Josh, and Mason, Libby and Jeff's sons, were always near with a hug and smile, and Mary and David's girls, Samantha and Andrea, stayed by my side.

Bill's friends warmed our hearts at the service held in First Baptist Church in Pflugerville. A group of SMA friends attended the service, including those who visited in the hospital: Delonda Delony; Jeff Price and his wife; Jeff McCord; Steve McCoy; Bobby Plyler; Brian Replogle; Caryl Toeppich Johnson and her mother, Carolyn Toeppich; Mike Draper, a pallbearer, and his mother, Virginia Thielepape; Lisa Bardwell; Scott Stewart;

Willie Vasquez and his wife; Dr. Jimmy Cobb, campus minister and Bible teacher at SMA; and Shella Baccus, business and English teacher. There were others unknown to me from SMA and friends Bill knew at work, as well as church friends who supported his family. Those unable to come called or sent their love over the Internet, by mail, and through beautiful floral offerings. God's men and women, who supported Bill in prayer, comforted our family.

Friends from Gore and Dell sustained him in untold ways during his struggle with cancer and comforted the family. Dell friends presented Bill with a blanket covered in sports emblems he highly prized, which is now a treasure for his family.

Mike Draper's mother, Virginia Thielepape, came in love for visitation. Randolph Beck, his wife, Eileen, and Lori Roeckers, from WORDsearch, were of great comfort to me the night of visitation.

In answer to my prayer in 2008, the Lord not only provided a Christian mentor for Bill, he provided friends at WORDsearch who gave to Bill immeasurably. I was overcome with the Lord's care of Bill and the support of WORDsearch in answer to my two-year-old prayer for a Christian mentor. WORDsearch supported Bill in every way imaginable, which included flexible work hours during chemo treatments. WORDsearch employees gave financial gifts to Bill, and WORDsearch matched their employees' funds.

Paul Petropolis, founder of Angels in Action, and his wife, Susan, drove from Houston to Bill's house to embrace me with love, letting me know how much they cared.

In a back room of the church with the family, I didn't see all of those who came to Bill's services, but Betty and Bob Driver, Yo Kawamoto, Carolyn Lacy, Lori and Jim Robertson, Julia and

David Todd, and Katie Todd (Austin), Reverend Larry Womack from Copperfield Church, and Isabel Piedrahita from Houston were among those I did see the day of the funeral. Our family came from Kentucky, Mississippi, Tennessee, and Texas.

At the service, Bill's pastor, Reverend Steve Washburn, witnessed to the loving grace of God and everlasting life. After the service, several individuals asked how to become a part of the Christian faith.

"Bill would have liked that," Carrie said.

Church friends hosted a bountiful buffet at the church for Bill's family and friends. A few tears were shed, but many smiles graced faces as we celebrated the life and home-going of our beloved, kindhearted, sweet loved one. Bill meant a lot to many. We wanted to remember the laughter and joy he brought to all of us.

Bill was acquainted with death and the glories of heaven through Scripture and sermons he'd heard. A Christmas before Bill's encounter with cancer, Bill and Carrie gave the book, *90 Minutes in Heaven*, by Don Piper, coauthored with Cecil Murphy, as gifts. This book about a Baptist minister in the presence of the glories of heaven intrigued Bill. He excitedly discussed the author's experience with me. Knowing Bill read *90 Minutes in Heaven* comforted me, for it gave him a glimpse of the magnificence of heaven.

Four months before the Lord took Bill, we were bystanders at the large funeral service at my old church in Kansas City. We visited the national cemetery in Leavenworth and President Truman and the First Lady's graves in Independence. In March 2010, I attended funeral services for Kitsy Campbell, my great-niece.

Was the Lord preparing us for the day Bill entered eternal life? I don't know. But I do know His love filled the church during Bill's service. People in a long line of cars, shepherded by four policemen on motorcycles, joined the family at the cemetery in Pflugerville. We celebrated our loved one's life and life everlasting in the service at the cemetery and at the luncheon. We were at peace knowing that Jesus cherished our beloved Bill, who was an inspiration and showed us the way to live more closely in God's will.

All souls are extraordinary. In God's loving arms, souls are extraordinary forever.

"And the rain descended, and the floods came, and the winds blew, and beat upon that house; and it fell not: for it was founded upon a rock" (Matthew 7:25).

Chapter Fourteen
God's DNA

I've wondered what it was in Bill that gave him the love and support of so many people. It wasn't charisma, though he had plenty of that. At first, I thought it was Bill's grace. Then I knew it was God's grace, a translucence of Him that others saw in Bill, the same translucence I'd seen in my toddler years ago in a Florida setting sun.

Modest and humble in manner with a multi-faceted heart stretched wide in tenderness and compassion, Bill won the race of life. At six feet, he was massive in stature. He rarely threw his weight around, but he could. Tough, cool, casual, and quick, our son looked out for the little guys. Bobby Plyler, his friend, called him God's giant. Bill gave God credit for who he was. "I will praise thee; for I am fearfully and wonderfully made: marvelous are thy works; and that my soul knoweth right well" (Psalm 139:14).

At the service, Bill's pastor, Reverend Steve Washburn of First Baptist Church in Pflugerville, mentioned that Bill was a giant of a man. While Bill was on chemo, I learned that he'd provided funds for someone he thought needy.

I was quick to criticize his kindness, "Those people are healthy. Let them figure out how to supply their own needs," I'd said.

"They have issues I don't have," Bill quickly countered.

Bill believed cancer wasn't the only knockout in life. His perception, a God-given intelligence and caring heart served the issues of others in circumstances that Bill considered more overwhelming than his battle with cancer. "Keep thy heart with all diligence; for out of it are the issues of life" (Proverbs 4:23).

Bill's relationship to his Master surfaced throughout his life. Friends saw his Maker's energy and steadfastness. God's gift of perception intensified Bill's innermost spirit, and others recognized his Master's power to simplify and solve problems, to see the true feelings and needs of others. Friends and family felt his Savior's gentle touch and love. Through a memorable resonance in dialogue, they heard his Redeemer's voice. Our Savior shone from within our son, and his long intimacy with Jesus beamed into our hearts. Bill's intelligence, strength, and confidence were God's DNA within him. "Which was the son of Enos, which was the son of Seth, which was the son of Adam, which was the son of God" (Luke 3:38).

God's DNA is replicated, infused into all of us before we are even formed in the womb. Before conception, God knew Bill and endowed him with an innermost being, an indescribable gift. God gloriously wrapped the treasure of His Spirit, secured it with a ribbon of choice, and boldly attached a badge of honor inscribed with Bill's name. Bill read the gift card, chose to unravel the ribbon, and opened God's present. He set free God's boundless love, and God's plan for his life to witness, and this witness will continue through his family and friends for generations to come. "Before I formed thee in the belly I knew thee; and before thou camest out of the womb I sanctified thee, and I ordained thee a prophet unto nations" (Jeremiah 1:5).

We won't forget Bill, his head high and shoulders thrust back, confidently striding about town, to work, and through the portals of church to take his seat in the sanctuary.

"You can't go to church, Bill," I recall saying. "You're just out of the hospital."

"I'm going to church, Mom. I don't want anyone to get my seat."

Bill never appeared to be aware of the bearing his voice and stature had on others, but he generated a presence every time he walked through a door. I cannot speak for God. But in a unique and lovable way, I believe God sanctified and ordained Bill to witness.

No man is perfect, and so it was with Bill. No one would take away his penchant to enjoy each day and his faith in God's will. He didn't hold grudges. He paddled his own canoe with God's hands on the paddles and, gliding along, witnessed God's redeeming grace and mercy. Our beloved reached for the stars in his faith, his family, and his work. He reached higher because he knew God.

Bill had great plans to be a part of the sales team at WORDsearch. He planned a return trip with Carrie to Germany. The Lord scheduled Bill's next trip, the most exciting, magnificent journey ever, passage paid—to eternity.

Chapter Fifteen
Eternity

Only God could have created the Bill we knew. We will never forget his sunny disposition, his sense of humor, quick wit, and enthusiasm for life. He was lively. He was resilient and loyal. I believe the qualities with which we identify Bill live with him amid heavenly splendors.

Bill's purpose in life on Earth was God given. He won't and doesn't want to re-enter Earth's realm. He left us with his faith in Christ. He never seemed consumed with fear. He never appeared embittered. He had a plan. He knew where he was going.

Who understands the magnificent power of communication in and from eternity? I can envision heavenly cell phones and chips and computers, in designs unfathomable to the human brain.

On Earth, God's Word, written by men inspired by God, inspired Bill. He tapped out Scripture on his laptop in e-mails to others. I can picture Bill busy and excited in heaven, working heavenly phones and tapping away on holy computers of God's design, beyond human imagination. After a heavenly workday, if there are Harleys in heaven, Bill's on one, zipping along on streets of gold or in his favorite NASCAR race car, racing around heaven's fastest track.

In thinking about Bill, I can almost hear, "This is Bill Roddy, Eternity. I met Him! I met Him face to face. Oh, the glory! You wouldn't believe this place. Man, this is the greatest! Unbelievable! You've got to come up here. I don't want you to miss it. Don't wait to get your ticket. Jesus paid for it in advance. Get it now! Be ready to come!"

Bill left his business card on the tablets of our hearts.

E T E R N I T Y

William Baine Roddy

Believe: John 3:16

Contact: Your local church

JesusChrist_24/7@UntoMe.come

Chapter Sixteen
Amid Heavenly Splendors

Carrie placed an imposing double marker on Bill's grave. Carved across the top of the monument is the name Roddy. Underneath the family name are open pages of the Holy Bible. Carrie is inscribed across the pages of the Bible on the right, and Bill's name etched on the pages of the Bible on the left. Tears welled in my eyes when I saw the marker. It wasn't the first time I'd seen a "B" and three sticks written across the pages of a Bible, recalling Bill's earliest signature scribbled across pages of our family Bible.

Beneath the Bible on the marker, John 11:25-26 is cut into the granite, "I am the resurrection and the life, he that believeth in me, though he were dead, yet shall he live. And whosoever liveth and believeth in me shall never die. Believest thou this!"

Bill lives amid heavenly splendors. John Parker, Bill's first pastor, reminded us if we want to see Bill again, we need to be ready to meet our Savior.

People offered expressions of sympathy, "Don't you know his grandparents hugged him?" And, "I know Bill's dad was excited to see him in heaven." The thoughts were comforting. Steve and Bill were full of enthusiasm.

It is easy to believe Steve met Bill with a big smile, "How's my boy?"

And Bill answering, with his blue eyes shining, "I can't believe this. Thanks, Dad, for the directions to get here."

★ ★ ★

As I pondered this heavenly scene, I came across a paragraph written by my husband on aging.

> One of the two recent examples I've encountered (verses related to aging) is John 9:5. The key word here is *light*. Light is made of bundles of photons traveling at 670 million miles per hour (or 186,000 miles per second). Nothing else travels this fast, but at that speed, time stops. Aging of everything stops and an eternal dimension is entered. What Jesus was saying is that He was light not only that we can see with our eyes, but that wherever He is, there is eternal.

★ ★ ★

To those of you who follow Racing:

WOW! Bill left here in an instant—at more than 670 million miles per hour (or 186,000 miles per second). In a twinkling of an eye, he was in eternity. Don't miss the fastest track ever. Believe. Jesus is waiting for you.

Bill's ambition since his first go-kart was to meet NASCAR drivers. August 2010, he planned to be in Bristol, Tennessee/ Virginia, for the NASCAR races and maybe realize his ambition. By August 2010, he'd met his Savior and was with Him in timeless heaven. He left a gift for his children to observe the earthly men he greatly admired, NASCAR drivers active in Motor Racing Outreach. With the NASCAR tickets, hotel reservations, and plane tickets that Bill bought early in the year, Carrie traveled with Amanda and Christopher to the NASCAR races at Bristol in August, 2010.

To SMA Alumni:

I can imagine when Jesus gathered Bill in His arms, Bill threw his arms around His Savior in a Bear (mascot) hug. They had been bonded for years. Jesus is waiting for a Bear hug from you. Don't miss eternity. Believe. Touchdown in heaven.

To Howard Payne University Alumni:

HPU reinforced Bill's belief in Jesus, and he found his beloved Carrie there. Teach your children to love the Lord, and they will believe too.

To Carrie, Christopher, and Amanda:

Bill loved you with all his heart and left you in His hands. I know you will never forget how good God is to us. Be happy and live your life for Him. You know the best is to come. Bill knew your abiding faith in Christ, and that you will witness for Him. Your witness will last for generations to come.

★   ★   ★

Libby and Mary and their families:

Bill lit up our hearts. We give thanks and praise to our Savior for Bill being a part of our lives. We will see Bill again. We will continue Bill's witness that will last for generations. We believe in a living Savior.

Bill's life on Earth witnesses to us now and forever in the name of the Father, the Son, and the Holy Spirit. Bill's witness to his faith lives; the fruit of his witness will never die. Wherever He is, there is the eternal; and Bill is with his Savior.

★   ★   ★

In the kitchen at my sink, I wind the steeple of the little copper church and hear "Amazing Grace" with a depth of emotion never before felt.

My prayer for you.

> Who also declared unto us your love in the Spirit.
> For this cause we also, since the day we heard it,
> do not cease to pray for you, and to desire that ye
> might be filled with the knowledge of his will in all
> wisdom and spiritual understanding; that ye might
> walk worthy of the Lord unto all pleasing, being
> fruitful in every good work, and increasing in the
> knowledge of God (Colossians 1:8-10). In Jesus'
> name. Amen.

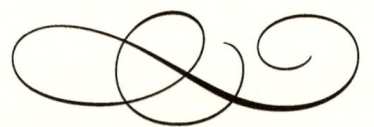

Chapter Seventeen
In the Pit:
Before Fifty, At Fifty, After Fifty

My son's fervor about prevention, early screening, a cure for cancer, and my own strong feelings over his untimely death in 2010 motivated the writing of this last chapter. I'd be remiss if I didn't share Bill's take on cancer and the spiraling financial costs of treating it. He dramatized the cost with a humorous monologue.

"When I walk in to get chemo, I'm greeted with a smile and hear, 'Hello-o-o, Mr. Roddy,' and the receptionist extends her hand for money. Think of the money spent for chemo. Money needs to go for early screening and finding a cure for cancer. Someone out there has a cure, but they are not getting the money to pull it together and market it. If Gore and Dell researched and WORDsearch published it, prevention, early screening, and a cure for cancer would close those chemo places down."

It may not be quite that simple, but Bill had a direct manner. He was fiercely competitive and believed in the know-how and technology of American companies. For those with cancer, chemotherapy is a life-saver and a holding pattern. Don't ever give up the fight. There is a cure out there.

An article in the *Smithsonian*, May 2011, "The Triumph of Dr. Druker," by Terence Monmaney, addresses concerns similar to Bill's about the cost of chemotherapy and shutting down cancer for patients as we know it today. In the article about Dr. Brian Druker, Oregon Health & Science University (OHSU), Portland, Oregon, Monmaney relates the story of Dr. Druker's success in developing a pill that has extended the lives of patients with chronic myeloid leukemia (CML), a blood cancer.

Scientists like Dr. Druker work tirelessly to defeat the disease. Knight Cancer Institute, established by Phil and Penny Knight at OHSU, with their contribution of $100 million, supports research to close the door on cancer. We need more research and tailor-made treatment for cancer victims. Physicians and biochemists work long hours researching possible cures for cancer. Continued financial support is critical for research scientists dedicated to obliterating colon cancer and all types of cancer.

Medical scientists are on track, but there are crucial laps to run. In the meantime, early screening renders hope to patients with colon polyps that become cancerous and can metastasize to major organs in the body.

It concerns me that men and women in the thirty-to-forty age range and the fifty-above group walk around with asymptomatic polyps or potential colon cancers. Sometime between Bill's thirty-fifth and forty-fifth years, he slipped through the cracks with a polyp that developed into colon cancer. My husband performed colon cancer surgery. I'd had two experiences with possible colon cancer before Bill's diagnosis with the dreaded disease. Our family was on the edge of a wealth of information about colon cancer. I've asked myself, *How could it happen?*

The average mother does not have a doctorate degree and license to practice motherhood, yet we deal with theology, education, and health issues daily. I know nothing more about cancer than I did about Bill's life at work. I have no experience in medicine. My children wouldn't let me put a Band-Aid® on them. I offer cradle advice, motherly advice garnered within the classroom experience of rearing a family, and my own medical history.

The study of preventing and finding a cure for cancer, understanding a complex abnormal division of cells in the body, happens in laboratories housed in multistoried buildings in major medical centers and with physicians who diagnose and treat cancer patients. The question gnawed away in my mind, *Could I have done anything in the children's early years that may have helped ward off Bill's cancer?* The answer, of course, is yes. I could have done better in my laboratory—the home. I should have been aware of what more a mother could do.

"Eat the vegetables on your plate. You've had your quota for sweets and junk food today." And, "Take a bath, brush, and floss your teeth. Go to bed. You need eight hours sleep tonight and every night. Did you have a bowel movement today? Yesterday? Regularity may help prevent colon cancer."

In answer to my own questions, I reviewed books and websites for information on risk factors and prevention. My research centered on major cancer centers associated with medical schools in the United States, and I found major cancer centers offered websites with excellent information on prevention and risk factors and the diagnosis and treatment of colorectal cancer.

Mayo Clinic offered a website on prevention. For information on prevention, I found www.mayoclinic.com/health/cancer-prevention/CA00024, and Mayo Clinic website that included dental hygiene and overall health, www.mayoclinic.com/health/dental/DE00001.

Fighting cancer or disease in the home and reviewing the best health habits, day in and day out, increases potential for better health. Parents need to be conscious of risk factors in colon cancer and monitor nutrition and the health habits of children and themselves as carefully as a captain of a ship monitors his vessel in a fog.

In researching risk considerations for colon cancer, I read cancer in other members of the family to be a factor. Accessing family medical history may not be easy in today's world of scattered, dysfunctional, and blended families, and lack of family medical history becomes a risk factor for colon cancer. Poor nutrition, lack of exercise and the use of tobacco and alcohol are risk factors in colon cancer. Diets high in fat, low in vegetables, contribute to poor nutrition, a risk factor in colon cancer. Sources studied recommended the age of fifty for initial colon cancer screening, however, risk factors add up and colon cancer screening may be advised before fifty.

According to M. D. Anderson House Call, Patient Information Sheet, risk factors establish who should be screened and how often. For further information review, The University of Texas M.D.Anderson House Call, Patient Information Sheet. "Colon Cancer Screening, Risk factors determine who should be screened." Posted September 2011. *Oncolog*, September

2011, Vol. 56, No.9. www2.mdanderson.org/depts/oncolog/
articles/11/9-sep/9-11-hc.html.

Colonoscopy is not the only examination for colorectal
cancer. MD Anderson's website offered screening guidelines for
colorectal exams. For further review of types of screening see,
University of Texas MD Anderson Cancer Center. "Colorectal
Cancer Screening Exams." Posted Year 2011. *Cancer Information*.
www.mdanderson.org/patient-and-cancer-information/cancer-
information/cancer-topics/prevention-and-screening/cancer-
screening-guidelines/colorectal-cancer-screening-exams.html.

Our body is our vehicle on Earth and needs attention.
Manufacturers do a great job marketing books, clothes, foods,
and vehicles for children and adults. Products come with care
instructions. We check batteries, carburetors, belts, hoses, and
tires on a car. If a red light pops up on the dash, we're off to a
mechanic. A car sputters and quits from flawed gasoline; a plane
crashes from bad fuel. Bad eating habits prove disastrous down
the road. An awareness of specific red flags, health-wise, may help
ward off colon cancer and other diseases months or years later.

Symptoms researched for colorectal cancer covered a
range of none and/or vague to obvious indications. According
to New York-Presbyterian Hospital's website there may be
warning signs with changes in bowel habits. NYPH offers
further information on their website, New York-Presbyterian
Hospital. "Digestive Diseases, Symptoms of Colorectal Cancer."
Clinical Services. www.nyp.org/services/digestive/colorectal-
cancer-symptoms.html. Another NYPH Website defines and
presents insight into colorectal cancer, New York-Presbyterian
Hospital.

Another descriptive text about colon cancer appeared at "Cancer, Colorectal, What is colorectal cancer?" Posted November 30,2008. *Health Library.* www.nyp.org/health/digest-colorectal.html.

It is easy to ignore vague symptoms in children and in ourselves. I ignored subtle digestive symptoms at age twenty-eight and again in 2008. With vague and repetitive colon problems, i.e., upset stomachs, do not self-diagnose, or take over-the-counter remedies, take someone else's medicine, or listen to do-gooders. Seek professional advice. Don't put off medical checkups.

It is handy to keep your own medical records. Request medical records each time you see a physician and for laboratory tests, X-rays, MRIs, sonograms, or anything else a doctor orders. This saves time if more medical evaluation is needed.

If diagnosed with a condition, mass, or symptom of cancer, seek a second opinion at a major cancer center as soon as possible. Don't wait. It is okay to ask the doctor who makes the initial diagnosis for an immediate referral for a second opinion or to call the closest cancer center for an appointment. If possible, go to one of the highest-ranking cancer hospitals for an evaluation and second opinion.

U. S. News & World Report, U.S. News Best Hospitals (2011-2012), surveyed nearly ten thousand specialists and compiled data for almost five thousand hospitals to rank the top hospitals in sixteen adult specialties. The honor roll features the top hospitals, including hospitals for cancer and gastroenterology. For further rankings, see *U.S. News & World Report.* "U.S. News Best Hospitals: Top Ranked Hospitals for Cancer." *U.S. News Health,* www. health.usnews.com/best-hospitals/rankings.

Physicians in foremost cancer hospitals have the advantage of information from thousands of cases and a store of statistics. Major cancer centers update information daily on the treatment and medicine best suited for each new case of cancer. If highly qualified gastroenterologists and oncologists are on your case from the beginning, they offer their expertise to you and to your referring physician. A second opinion is in the best interest of the patient. Medical records in hand cuts time with an appointment for a second opinion consultation.

Gastroenterology is the study of diseases from the mouth through the digestive tract to the anus. A board-certified gastroenterologist is the physician qualified for advice or for treatment of digestive problems. For top ranked gastroenterology hospitals, see U.S. New & World Report. "U.S. News Best Hospitals: Doctors: Gastroenterology." *U.S. News Health,* www. health.usnews.com/besthospitals/rankings/digestive-disorders.

Colon polyps may be present ten years before colon cancer is discovered. In the 1960s, my husband, Stephen R. Roddy, MD, FACS, addressed the problem in a talk on colon cancer at a local meeting of the American Cancer Society at St. Joseph's Hospital, Port Charlotte, Florida. In the speech, he emphasized early detection of polyps that can become cancerous. The following is an excerpt from his talk:

The average age of a patient with adenomatous polyps is ten years less than that for actual cancer. Wider resections done by surgeons have increased the number of patients cured, but earlier diagnosis remains the *key essential element* in successful treatment of colon cancer.

Dr. Roddy's speech included interesting historical references. As early as 1296, surgical intervention for bowel problems was recognized by Lanfranc of Milan. Lanfranc's treatise showed up in Guy de Chauliac's *Chirurgia Magna* or *Great Surgery*, first printed in Venice in 1490. Guy de Chauliac was a physician and surgeon foremost in his day. In 1826, Lambert described a method of sewing, or suturing, the bowel back together or approximating the ends of the bowel in a procedure called anastomosis. The references to colon surgery were found on:

> www.en.wikipedia.org/wiki/Lanfranc_of_Milan,
> www.en.wikipedia.org/wiki/Guy_de_Chauliac
> www.en.wikipedia.org/wiki/Antoine Lembert.

Anastomosis of the colon was a giant step forward in colon surgery, but doomed until physicians had access to medicines to control infections. During the twentieth century, the cure rate for colon surgery advanced impressively.

In Dr. Roddy's 1965 speech, he stated that in 1925 the French Surgical Congress summarized all the accomplishments in colon surgery up to that time. The five-year cure rate in 1925 for colon surgery was ten percent. In 1965, the cure rates ranged from 52 percent to 92 percent. Stephen R. Roddy, MD, FACS. "Review of *Colon Cancer*" (presentation before the American Cancer Society, St. Joseph's Hospital, Port Charlotte, Florida, 1965).

According to anchor Katie Couric on the NBC *Today* show if detected early, patients with colon cancer had a ninety percent cure rate. For reference see Katie Couric, Anchor: "Confronting Colon Cancer, I must share this vital information." NBC, "Today". Updated March 31, 2004, 1:44:48 PM ET, New York: 2004. http://today.msnbc.msn.com/id/4602812/ns/today/t/katie-couric-i-must-share-vital-information/ (Accessed February 17, 2012). See references,

Gorman, Christine. "Katie's Crusade." *Time* 155, no. 10 (March 13, 2000) or Gorman, Christine. Katie's Crusade, Cover Story, ©Time Magazine. (2002):1-6, e-document.

According to an article in the *American Journal of Gastroenterology*, 1989 September; 84, No. 9, by W. I. Wolff and the Department of Surgery, Beth Israel Medical Center in New York, utilizing advances with the development of the colonoscope and endoscope, physicians were able to view the colon in its entirety. Viewing the colon in its entirety dramatically increased the detection and excision of polyps in the colon. It took centuries to realize a colon cancer cure rate of ninety percent.

A ninety percent cure rate for colon cancer if detected early is the positive news, but in the twenty-first century, colon cancer persists in thousands of people. According to the American Cancer Society's Explore Research/ Cancer Facts & Figures 2012, page 4, estimated new Cases, male and female, U. S., 2012, page 4 were:

103,130 new cases of colon cancer
40, 290 new cases of rectal cancer
6,230 anal cases

According to the American Cancer Society's, Explore Research/Cancer Facts & Figures 2012, estimated deaths, U.S., for colorectal cancers, U.S., page 6, were:

51,690

For further reading, American Cancer Society, www.cancer.org/ acs/groups/content/@epidemiologysurveilance/documents/

document/acspc-031941.pdf and American Cancer Society's "Estimated Deaths, U.S., 2012." Explore Research/Cancer Facts & Figures 2012, page 6. *Explore Research/ Cancer Facts & Figures.*

www.cancer.org/acs/groups/content/@epidemiology surveilance/documents/document/acspc-031941.pdf.
American Cancer Society's. "Estimated New Cases, Male and Female, U. S., 2012." Posted Year 2012, page 4. *Explore Research/ Cancer Facts & Figures.*
www.cancer.org/acs/groups/content/@epidemiology surveilance/documents/document/acspc-031941.pdf.

The problem today (2012) is getting patients in for any type of colon screening that includes colonoscopy before fifty, at fifty, and after fifty. Internet sources reveal the value of early screening for colon cancer on websites of major cancer centers. According to the New York-Presbyterian Hospital website, patients may or may not experience symptoms that relate to colorectal cancer. Vague digestive symptoms may be warning signs for other colon problems or other health issues. Among the websites researched at New York Presbyterian Hospital for symptoms and screening were: New York-Presbyterian Hospital. *Digestive Diseases, Symptoms of Colorectal Cancer. Clinical Services.* www.nyp.org/services/digestive/colorectal-cancer-symptoms.html. and New York-Presbyterian Hospital News. "Make That Call for Colon Cancer Screening: It Could Save Your Life." Posted March 1, 2011. *Katie Couric, NYC Department of Health and WCBS-TV Launch Citywide Campaign. New York Presbyterian Hospital Jan Monahan Center.* www.nyp.org/news/hospital/colon-cancer-screening-couric.html.

In my experience, only a clinician can accurately diagnose colorectal cancer. Unusual or abnormal gastrointestinal problems present in any age group, child or adult, need to be reviewed by a gastroenterologist. Seek second opinions for continued vague, unexplained symptoms. If tests for symptoms of colon cancer are negative and vague abdominal symptoms persist, seek the opinion of other board-certified specialists. If you are a woman, ask for the advice of a gynecologist. Take charge of your own health.

I ignored vague symptoms that could have cost my life. There are references in medical literature of my experience at twenty-eight that detail the obstruction of the colon and subsequent surgery. (See Harwell Wilson, M.D., *Annals of Surgery*, Volume 151, no. 6, June 1960, p. 910.) In 2008, I again ignored vague symptoms that continued until a physician ordered a colonoscopy, and then I postponed it. When the colonoscopy was done, physicians found a large precancerous polyp in the upper right colon. Fortunately, the polyp was removed before cancer cells took over.

Age fifty remains the standard for colon cancer screening. Bill's concern was preventing and finding colon polyps before they become cancerous at any age. According to an article by Christine Traxler, MD, "The Quest to Change Colon Cancer Screening," *Colon Cancer Resource News Issue,* no. 045, October 13, 2010, there is a need to change guidelines for earlier screening for colon cancer in the thirty-to-forty age group. For further information: Traxler, Christine. "The Quest to Change Colon Cancer Screening." *Colon Cancer Resource: Helping You Find a Cure.* no. 045. Posted October 13, 2010. *Colon Cancer Resource.* www.coloncancerresource.com/CCR_News-CCR News45.html.

Those who have brought colon cancer to the attention of the public are to be commended and highly praised. Tremendous efforts on the part of celebrities and the media to herald early screening for colon cancer to the public has saved lives. Occasional media spotlights about colon cancer are not sufficient. The potential of colon cancer in the general population is great and costly enough to warrant reminding the general population nonstop.

In my opinion, the general American public is unaware of the need for early screening for colon cancer before the age of fifty, at fifty, and after fifty. Highly visible reminders of the dangers of colon cancer-related symptoms and the need for an awareness of the vague symptoms of colon cancer don't exist in places frequented by active men and women. Symptoms and screening for colon cancer advertised in sites common to busy working individuals would be an avenue to acquaint the general public with the perils of colon cancer. Posters placed in employee lounges, sports and entertainment arenas, pharmacy and grocery stores, and hospitals would alert potential victims of colon cancer.

ALERT!
BEFORE FIFTY, AT FIFTY, AND AFTER FIFTY
AN AWARENESS OF PREVENTION AND RISK
FACTORS FOR COLON CANCER
SAVES LIVES
DO YOU KNOW YOUR RISK FACTORS?

Families of colorectal cancer victims endure heartache and financial upheavals when a family member is diagnosed with colon cancer, and the family may be a significant factor in pushing for research of colorectal cancer. We need a public push for new lines of thought for prevention and screening for colon cancer—before fifty, at fifty, and after fifty.

The last mile in a race to win may be the hardest, and the last stretch to beat colon cancer may be the most difficult, and require the most effort and financing. Doctors and scientists dedicated to preventing, treating, and finding a cure for cancer need our encouragement and financial support.

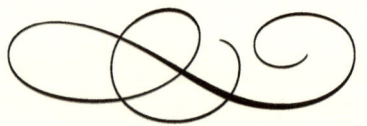

Epilogue

During WWII, the United States military created the 5307th Composite Unit, a special unit under General Frank Merrill, to fight overwhelming odds. In slightly more than five months, behind Japanese enemy lines, the 5307th Unit advanced 750 miles through some of the harshest jungle terrain in the world, fought in five major engagements, and engaged in combat with the Japanese army on thirty-two separate occasions. They often fought an unseen enemy. Their achievement astounded military and non-military alike.

WWII Merrill's Marauders survivors and descendants banded together to honor buddies and family members injured or killed in battle and by disease and hunger, by keeping alive the memory and sacrifices of their loved ones. The valiant effort of the Merrill's Marauders may be found at the Center of Military History and Wikipedia's websites.

Center of Military History, United States Army. "Merrill's Marauders." American Forces in Action Series. 1945. Washington, DC: *CMH Publications 100-104*, 1945

www.history.army.mil/books/wwii/marauders/ marauders-fw.htm and Wikipedia Free Encyclopedia. "Merrill's Maruaders." Modified December 24, 2011. *Wikipedia Foundation, Inc.* www.en.wikipedia.org/wiki/Merrill's_Marauders.

The historical significance of Merrill's Marauders, men who faced insurmountable odds and never gave up, continues to inspire us today. Their dedication to win is what we need to fight colon cancer and all cancer.

Our lost ones did not fall in military battle. Ravaged by an enemy seen only on colonoscopies, CAT scans, and MRIs, similar to images seen with nighttime binoculars on a battlefield, our loved ones fought colon cancer in rooms off hospital corridors.

The medical community has made great strides in detecting colon polyps and in surgical excision of polyps that can become cancerous. The battle won't be victorious without the dedication and tremendous efforts of scientists and volunteers of healthy men and women who want to win over colon cancer or any cancer. We are not there yet.

In my reading about colon cancer and cancer in general, I found endless possibilities for young scientists to pursue the doom of cancer. America offers the environment for students to realize dreams in medical science that will become a reality and offer hope to patients with cancer.

Education and funding for colon/colorectal cancer, the second leading cause of cancer-related deaths for men and women combined, is grave. With a mighty drive from volunteers and financial support for early screening and research, scientists can raise the survival statistics for colon cancer victims and all cancer victims.

The end is in sight. Let's put our shoulders to the grindstone and synchronize our energy. It's what Americans do best, you know. Support early screening for colon cancer and help win the race with all cancers.

The Pirate won't win,
Prevention and
Early screening will knock
Polyp out of the park.
Family and friends the world over
Honor our loved ones Brave and
In God's will,
Others will be saved.

References

American Cancer Society's. "Estimated Deaths, U.S., 2012."
Explore Research/Cancer Facts & Figures." Posted Year 2012,
page 6. *Explore Research/ Cancer Facts & Figures.* www.cancer.
org/acs/groups/content/@epidemiologysurveilance/
documents/document/acspc-031941.pdf.
(Accessed January 9, 2012.)

American Cancer Society's. "Estimated New Cases, Male and
Female, U. S., 2012." Posted Year 2012, page 4. *Explore
Research/ Cancer Facts & Figures.* www.cancer.org/acs/
groups/content/@epidemiologysurveilance/documents/
document/acspc-031941.pdf. (Accessed January 9, 2012)

Berger, Eric. "Supercomputer to benefit Rice, Medical Center,
IBM supercomputer to benefit Rice, Medical Center."
Houston and Texas News, *Houston Chronicle.* March 1, 2010.
www.chron.com/disp/story.mpl/metropolitan/6892273.
html. (Accessed January 25, 2011.)

Branley, Franklyn Mansfield. *The Christmas Sky.* New York, NY:
Thomas Y. Crowell, 1966.

Branley, Franklyn Mansfield. *The Christmas Sky.* New York, NY:
Thomas Y. Crowell, 1990.

Center of Military History, United States Army. *Merrill's Marauders*. American Forces in Action series. Washington, DC: CMH Publications, 1945.

Couric, Katie. "Confronting Colon Cancer, I must share this vital information." NBC, "Today". Updated March 31, 2004, 1:44:48 PM ET. New York: 2004. http://today.msnbc.msn.com/id/4602812/ns/today/t/katie-couric-i-must-share-vital-information/ (Accessed February 17, 2012).

Crick, Denal, and Diane Heard. *The Crest, 66*, San Marcos Baptist Academy, San Marcos, Texas. San Angelo, Texas: Newsfoto Yearbooks, 1981.

Gorman, Christine. "Katie's Crusade." *Time* 155, no. 10 (March 13, 2000).

Gorman, Christine. Katie's Crusade, Cover Story. *Time Magazine*. (2002):1-6, e-document.

Mayo Clinic Staff. *Staying Healthy "Cancer prevention: 7 tips to reduce your risk"*, Mayo Clinic; Posted September 21, 2010. www.mayoclinic.com/health/cancer-prevention/CA00024. (Accessed January 4, 2012.) (Accessed December 31, 2011.)

Monmaney, Terence. "The Triumph of Dr. Druker." *Smithsonian* (May 2011): 54-65.

New York-Presbyterian Hospital. "Cancer Screening and Prevention Colorectal Cancer." *Clinical Services*. www.nyp.org/services/digestive/colorectal-cancersymptoms.html (Accessed July 7, 2011.)

New York-Presbyterian Hospital. "Cancer, Colorectal, What is colorectal cancer?" Health Library; www.nyp.org/health/digest-colorectal.html November 30, 2008 (Accessed January 6, 2012.)

New York-Presbyterian Hospital. "Digestive Diseases, Symptoms of Colorectal Cancer." *Clinical Services* www.nyp.org/services/digestive/colorectal-cancer-symptoms.html (Accessed December 26, 2011.)

New York-Presbyterian Hospital News. "Make That Call for Colon Cancer Screening: It Could Save Your Life." Posted March 1, 2011. *Katie Couric, NYC Department of Health and WCBS-TV Launch Citywide Campaign. New York Presbyterian Hospital Jan Monahan Center.* www.nyp.org/news/hospital/colon-cancer-screening-couric.html. (Accessed December 10, 2011.)

Mayo Clinic. "Adult Health,Staying Health: Oral health: A window to your overall health," *Mayo Clinic Health Information.* www.mayoclinic.com/health/dental/DE00001 (Accessed December 31, 2011.)

Petropolis, Paul. "An Angel in Action." *Cy-Fair Magazine* (Summer 2011): 116-119.

Piper, Don, and Cecil Murphy. *90 Minutes in Heaven.* Grand Rapids, Michigan: Revell, 2004.

Roddy, Stephen R., MD, FACS. "Review of *Colon Cancer.*" (presentation before the American Cancer Society, St. Joseph's Hospital, Port Charlotte, FL, 1965).

Roddy, William B. "Bear Bryant" (unpublished *Journal of Poetry*, 1979).

————. "The Greatest Defeat" (unpublished *Journal of Poetry*, 1979).

————. "My Favorite Tree" (unpublished *Journal of Poetry*, 1979).

Roizen, Michael, MD, and Mehmet Oz, MD. "The You Docs: Health and Fitness. Your Anti Cancer Menu." *Houston Chronicle* (February 1, 2010): D4.

Jean Shand. *Echoes in Your Memories of San Marcos Baptist Academy.* San Marcos, Texas: Hays County Historical Commission, 1990.

Smith, Russell. "Seniors Shoulder Academy Load." *San Marcos Daily Record.* Oct. 4, 1981: 8A.

Standish, Burt L. *Frank Merriwell at Yale.* Whitefish, Montana: Kessinger Publishing, 2000.

Steimetz, Kriati A., PhD, RD, and John D. Potter, MD. "Vegetables, Fruit, and Cancer Prevention: A Review." *Journal of the American Diet Association* 96 (1996): 1027-1039.

Traxler, Christine. "The Quest to Change Colon Cancer Screening." *Colon Cancer Resource: Helping You Find a Cure.* no. 045. Posted October 13, 2010. *Colon Cancer Resource.* www.coloncancerresource.com/CCR_News-CCRNews45.html. (Accessed December 26, 2011)

The University of Texas MD Anderson Cancer Center. *"Screening for Colorectal Cancer"* Posted September 9, 2011. *Oncolog.* *www2.mdanderson.org/depts/oncolog/articles/11/9-sep/9-11-hc.html* (Accessed December 26, 2011.)

University of Texas MD Anderson Cancer Center. "Colorectal Cancer Screening Exams." Posted Year 2011. *Cancer Information.* www.mdanderson.org/patient-and-cancer-information/cancer-information/cancer-topics/prevention-and-screening/cancer-screening-guidelines/colorectal-cancer-screening-exams.html. (Accessed December 26, 2011.)

U.S. News & World Report. "U.S. News Best Hospitals: Top Ranked Hospitals for Cancer." Year 2012. *U.S. News Health.* www.health.usnews.com/best-hospitals/rankings/digestive-disorders. (Accessed January 10, 2012.)

U.S. New & World Report. "U.S. News Best Hospitals: Doctors: Gastroenterology." *U.S. News Health*. www. health.usnews. com/best-hospitals/rankings/digestive-disorders. (Accessed January, 10, 2012.)

Wikipedia. "Guy de Chauliac," modified October 17, 2011. Wikipedia Foundation. en.wikipedia.org/wiki/Guy de Chauliac. (Accessed December 26, 2011.) Wikipedia. "Lanfranc of Milan," modified December 24,2011. Originally, Lanfranc,Guido. *"Chirurgia Magna."* *Wikipedia Foundation, Inc.*www.en.wikipedia.org/wiki/Lanfranc_of_ Milan (Accessed December 26, 2011.)

Wikipedia. "Lembert's suture." Emerson, Ole Daniel. *Whonamedit? A dictionary of medical eponyms*. Originally published by A. Lembert. "Mémoire sur l'entéroraphie avec la descriptio d'un procédé nouveau pour pratiquer cette opération chirurgicale. Répertoire général d'anatomie et de physiologie pathologiques, Paris, 1826, 2: 10-107. (Accessed July 6, 2011.)

Wikipedia Free Encylopedia. "Merrill's Maruaders." Modified December 24, 2011. *Wikipedia Foundation, Inc.* www. en.wikipedia.org/wiki/Merrill's_Marauders. (Accessed January 10, 2012.)

Wilson, Harwell, MD. "Discussion." *Annals of Surgery* 151, no. 6 (June 1960): 910.

Wilson, Harwell, MD, and W. T. Tyson, MD. "Endometriosis in the Sigmoid Colon." *Mississippi Doctor* 31, no. 9 (February 1954): 297-9.

Wolff, W. I. "Colonoscopy: history and development." *American Journal of Gastroenterology* 84, no. 9 (September 1989): 1017-25.

Resources

These addresses may prove helpful in searching for guidelines regarding colon cancer:

American Board of Surgery, Inc.
1617 John F. Kennedy Blvd., Suite 860
Philadelphia, PA 19103
215) 568-4000

American Cancer Society, Inc.
American Cancer Society Guidelines on Nutrition and Physical
    Activity for Cancer
250 Williams Street, Suite. 600
Atlanta, Georgia 30303
Phone: 404-320-3333
Fax: 404-982-3677

American College of Gastroenterology
P.O. Box 342260
Bethesda, Maryland
301-263-9000.

Early detection and treatment is the number one assurance against colorectal cancer, and the best hope against its ravages.

After his diagnosis with colon cancer, Bill Roddy became outspoken and adamant about the need for early screening and funding for medical scientists. He heralded a mighty push for American corporate leadership to shut down cancer as we know it today.

In Bill's quest for new lines of thought for a cancer cure, he threw a mighty lance and tossed out God's streamers for others to catch and hold. Amid humor and chuckles and smiles, he left an extraordinary legacy of love and trust in God's will.

Join the author in sharing this book and its lessons with those you love and about whom you care. It's a gift of life that will keep on giving.

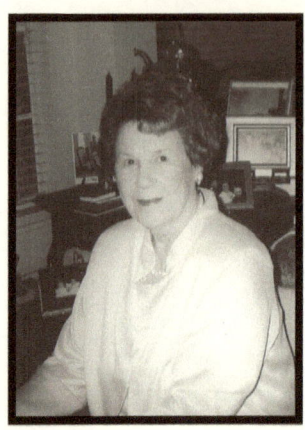

Martha Roddy and her surgeon husband reared their three children in Florida and Texas. She writes from a heart of Southern grace. Martha enjoys eight grandchildren and active memberships in the Society of Children's Book Writers and Illustrators and Inspirational Writers Alive! in Houston.

Notes